Nurses! Test Yourself in Essential Calculation Skills

Nurses! Test Yourself in . . .

Titles published in this series:

Nurses! Test Yourself in Anatomy and Physiology
Katherine M. A. Rogers and William N. Scott

Nurses! Test Yourself in Pathophysiology
Katherine M. A. Rogers and William N. Scott

Nurses! Test Yourself in Essential Calculation Skills
Katherine M. A. Rogers and William N. Scott

Visit www.mcgraw-hill.co.uk/openup/testyourself for further information
and sample chapters from other books in the series.

Nurses!
Test Yourself in
Essential Calculation
Skills

**Katherine M. A. Rogers and
William N. Scott**

McGraw Hill

Open University Press

Open University Press
McGraw-Hill Education
McGraw-Hill House
Shoppenhangers Road
Maidenhead
Berkshire
England
SL6 2QL

email: enquiries@openup.co.uk
world wide web: www.openup.co.uk

and Two Penn Plaza, New York, NY 10121-2289, USA

First published 2011

A catalogue record of this book is available from the British Library

ISBN-13: 978-0-33-524359-4
ISBN-10: 0335243592
eISBN: 978-0-33-524360-0

Library of Congress Cataloging-in-Publication Data
CIP data applied for

Typeset by RefineCatch Limited, Bungay, Suffolk
Printed in the UK by Bell & Bain Ltd, Glasgow

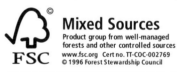

Mixed Sources
Product group from well-managed
forests and other controlled sources
www.fsc.org   Cert no. TT-COC-002769
© 1996 Forest Stewardship Council

The McGraw·Hill Companies

PRAISE FOR THIS BOOK

"This book will be of great benefit to student nurses. Following the clear, step by step guides and worked examples will enable you to quickly develop the confidence to master more complex processes. It will also be an invaluable resource for mentors supporting students."

Dorothy Adam, Lecturer, The Robert Gordon University, UK

"This book is a fundamental companion for all nurses wanting to become more proficient at medication calculations. The book is designed to find areas for improvements through a series of tests that start with a basic calculation review. Working through the book will help you to build confidence in the clinical environment."

James Pearson-Jenkins, Senior Lecturer of Adult Acute Nursing,
University of Wolverhampton, UK

"This book is a useful tool for all nurses. I would recommend it for nursing staff undertaking intravenous or other medication management courses/ modules. It would also benefit nurses who have to undertake calculations tests as part of their new post or ongoing development."

Amy Hutchinson, Student Nurse, University of Ulster, UK

"Through simple examples, exercises and gradual progression, this book will help to remove the anxiety often associated with the arithmetic involved in drug calculations commonly encountered in clinical practice. The book will be of use to pre-registration and registered nurses alike. It provides an opportunity for both self assessment and practice, as such it will be a useful tool for improving confidence, competence and patient safety in a critical skill."

Jim Jolly, Head of Academic Unit for Long Term Conditions,
School of Healthcare, University of Leeds, UK

Contents

Contents

Acknowledgements

We wish to thank Rachel Crookes, Claire Munce, Della Oliver and the rest of the team at McGraw-Hill-OUP for all their help and support throughout the writing of this text. We would also like to acknowledge all the reviewers who read our manuscript and provided us with very useful feedback.

About the authors

Dr. Katherine Rogers and Dr. William Scott are lecturers in applied health sciences with the School of Nursing and Midwifery at Queen's University Belfast where they teach health science subjects, including anatomy, physiology, pathophysiology and pharmacology to both undergraduate and postgraduate students of nursing science. They are also External Examiners in these subjects in a number of Higher Education Institutions across the UK.

Using this book

This book is designed to help you identify and address any potential weaknesses in your essential calculation skills. In turn this will help you become more confident and proficient in the aspects of numeracy that are an essential part of modern nursing care.

You may find an electronic calculator useful to check your answers, but remember that calculators may not always be available in the workplace, and that their use in clinical practice is generally discouraged. You need to become confident in applying calculation skills without the aid of a calculator.

The text is divided into two main sections. The first looks at basic calculation skills, and the second looks at some of the common calculation processes that nurses use. Each section includes two *diagnostic tests* designed to help you identify areas of concern. The book then directs you to specific worked examples that will guide you through the processes involved in successful calculation, so that you can understand each skill more fully, and master the art of successful calculation. Don't worry if you can't answer all of the questions in these tests, as your skills will improve with practice, and this book is designed to help you improve your skills!

If you systematically attempt each of the question areas your confidence in calculation skills will increase, making you a more proficient and safer practitioner. You may prefer to attempt only those areas that you currently have difficulty with, or which may be relevant in your own particular situation; the book is designed to allow you to 'dip in' to these specific areas.

You know best what you want to be able to accomplish with respect to your calculation skills. With practice, *Nurses! Test Yourselves in Essential Calculation Skills* can help you achieve this.

Abbreviations and symbols

cm	centimetre
g	gram
h	hour
IV	intravenous
kg	kilogram
L	litre
m	metre
mg	milligram
mL	millilitre
PEG	percutaneous endoscopic gastrostomy
NMC	Nursing and Midwifery Council
TI	therapeutic index
+	add
−	subtract
×	multiply
÷	divide
=	equals
%	percentage

SECTION A
Basic calculations review

INTRODUCTION

Many healthcare professionals are anxious when it comes to calculation skills, both in examination and in practice. Calculation skills can be a source of worry for many, and although the calculations you need in clinical situations are not always complex, they can be challenging when you are under pressure. Healthcare professionals need to be able to use numbers with confidence and safety, particularly when administering drugs.

Within the field of nursing, the importance of numeracy and calculation skills is emphasized by the fact that the Nursing and Midwifery Council (NMC) has recently changed the essential entry requirements for undergraduate courses to include proficiency in manipulating and utilizing numbers. Furthermore, the NMC now includes numeracy in its standards of proficiency, and requires students to undergo examination at two points within the nurse training programme.

This first section of the book tests your understanding of basic numeracy and calculation skills. The second section looks at specific areas of nursing practice that commonly use these number manipulations. This will enable you to assess your skills and see where you need to improve.

You should start by attempting all the questions in the *diagnostic test*, and then compare your answers with the ones given at the end of the test. If you find you've made consistent errors, you should read the appropriate chapter, which will give you specific help with that type of calculation.

For example, if you have problems with questions relating to *division*, you should go to the chapter that looks at division in greater detail. Then, when you are confident that you understand the approach to take, you should attempt the *check-up test* included at the end of the chapter. A second diagnostic test at the end of this first section will help you reassess your overall understanding of all these areas, and show how you have improved.

To get the most benefit from these tests, we suggest that an electronic calculator is used only to check your answers.

Remember, this text is designed primarily as a self-help resource for the most common areas of calculation that people have difficulty with. Some of the areas may seem trivial to you, but to someone else they may be a source of extreme concern and anxiety. Equally, other people may have no problem with areas that you find difficult.

Work through the areas that you have difficulty with at your own pace, and never be afraid to ask for help if there are areas that you continue to find difficult. Above all, be honest with yourself when checking your answers.

The essential thing to remember is that, if you use this text properly, it will help you become proficient in all these areas of calculation, making you a safer and more confident practitioner.

FOR EACH OF THE FOLLOWING CALCULATE THE CORRECT ANSWER

1 **Addition**

   a. 4 + 8   b. 6 + 9   c. 8 + 8

   d. 3 + 7   e. 5 + 6   f. 7 + 2

2 **Addition**

   a. 0.2 + 0.7   b. 0.4 + 0.8   c. 0.5 + 0.6

   d. 0.5 + 0.9   e. 0.8 + 0.7   f. 0.2 + 0.6

3 **Subtraction**

   a. 9 − 5   b. 4 − 3   c. 8 − 5

   d. 5 − 3   e. 7 − 4   f. 6 − 2

4 **Subtraction**

   a. 0.8 − 0.6   b. 0.5 − 0.4   c. 0.7 − 0.2

   d. 0.6 − 0.4   e. 0.9 − 0.2   f. 0.3 − 0.1

5 **Multiplication**
  a. 4×10 b. 6×10 c. 8×10

  d. 5×10 e. 7×10 f. 9×10

6 **Multiplication**
  a. 0.5×10 b. 0.7×10 c. 0.4×10

  d. 0.8×10 e. 0.3×10 f. 0.1×10

7 **Multiplication**
  a. 5×4 b. 6×3 c. 4×8

  d. 7×5 e. 3×8 f. 2×9

8 **Multiplication**
  a. 14×8 b. 11×4 c. 12×7

  d. 17×3 e. 15×6 f. 13×5

9 **Division**
  a. $3 \div 10$ b. $8 \div 10$ c. $5 \div 10$

  d. $4 \div 10$ e. $9 \div 10$ f. $6 \div 10$

10 **Division**
  a. $6.2 \div 10$ b. $9.8 \div 10$ c. $7.9 \div 10$

  d. $5.5 \div 10$ e. $4.1 \div 10$ f. $8.7 \div 10$

11 **Division**

    a. $8 \div 2$ b. $6 \div 3$ c. $9 \div 3$

    d. $5 \div 1$ e. $4 \div 2$ f. $8 \div 4$

12 **Division**

    a. $14 \div 2$ b. $18 \div 3$ c. $15 \div 3$

    d. $27 \div 9$ e. $28 \div 2$ f. $49 \div 7$

13 **Simplification**

    a. $\dfrac{4}{2}$ b. $\dfrac{6}{3}$ c. $\dfrac{6}{4}$

    d. $\dfrac{2}{6}$ e. $\dfrac{3}{9}$ f. $\dfrac{3}{18}$

14 **Simplification**

    a. $\dfrac{14}{2}$ b. $\dfrac{18}{3}$ c. $\dfrac{64}{8}$

    d. $\dfrac{2}{24}$ e. $\dfrac{24}{36}$ f. $\dfrac{6}{18}$

15 **Simplification**

    a. $\dfrac{400}{500}$ b. $\dfrac{350}{450}$ c. $\dfrac{320}{600}$

    d. $\dfrac{360}{300}$ e. $\dfrac{630}{540}$ f. $\dfrac{840}{720}$

16 **Simplification**

a. $\dfrac{0.4}{0.2}$ b. $\dfrac{0.6}{0.3}$ c. $\dfrac{0.8}{0.4}$

d. $\dfrac{0.4}{0.8}$ e. $\dfrac{0.2}{0.1}$ f. $\dfrac{0.9}{0.3}$

17 **Round to one decimal place**

a. 0.47 b. 0.89 c. 0.93

d. 1.24 e. 3.82 f. 4.55

18 **Round to two decimal places**

a. 5.877 b. 8.995 c. 6.327

d. 5.233 e. 3.755 f. 2.499

19 **Round to three decimal places**

a. 1.0166 b. 3.6832 c. 7.5554

d. 6.4338 e. 4.8326 f. 5.5555

20 **Change to improper fractions**

a. $2\dfrac{4}{5}$ b. $3\dfrac{7}{8}$ c. $5\dfrac{3}{4}$

d. $9\dfrac{2}{3}$ e. $8\dfrac{7}{9}$ f. $6\dfrac{1}{4}$

21 **Change to improper fractions**

a. $9\frac{11}{14}$ b. $7\frac{8}{13}$ c. $4\frac{10}{16}$

d. $6\frac{8}{27}$ e. $5\frac{6}{41}$ f. $8\frac{8}{29}$

22 **Change to mixed numbers**

a. $\frac{11}{4}$ b. $\frac{16}{7}$ c. $\frac{27}{6}$

d. $\frac{13}{5}$ e. $\frac{19}{8}$ f. $\frac{14}{3}$

23 **Change to decimal equivalents**

a. $\frac{3}{8}$ b. $\frac{4}{5}$ c. $\frac{1}{4}$

d. $\frac{3}{6}$ e. $\frac{3}{4}$ f. $\frac{6}{8}$

24 **Change to decimal equivalents**

a. $\frac{27}{30}$ b. $\frac{12}{24}$ c. $\frac{21}{84}$

d. $\frac{18}{90}$ e. $\frac{11}{44}$ f. $\frac{10}{80}$

25 **Convert the following volumes**
   a. 250 microlitres to millilitres
   b. 500 microlitres to millilitres
   c. 635 microlitres to millilitres
   d. 1.27 millilitres to microlitres
   e. 2.63 millilitres to microlitres
   f. 4.61 millilitres to microlitres

26 **Convert the following volumes**
   a. 100 millilitres to litres
   b. 240 millilitres to litres
   c. 825 millilitres to litres
   d. 0.5 litres to millilitres
   e. 0.64 litres to millilitres
   f. 0.785 litres to millilitres

27 **Convert the following weights**
   a. 200 milligrams to grams
   b. 375 milligrams to grams
   c. 950 milligrams to grams
   d. 0.4 grams to milligrams
   e. 0.55 grams to milligrams
   f. 0.684 grams to milligrams

28 **Convert the following weights**
   a. 120 grams to kilograms
   b. 250 grams to kilograms
   c. 588 grams to kilograms
   d. 0.2 kilograms to grams
   e. 0.45 kilograms to grams
   f. 0.825 kilograms to grams

29 **Express as a percentage**

    a. 0.25   b. 0.45   c. 0.95

    d. 0.27   e. 0.63   f. 0.47

30 **Express as a percentage**

    a. $\dfrac{1}{2}$ b. $\dfrac{3}{4}$ c. $\dfrac{4}{8}$

    d. $\dfrac{9}{10}$ e. $\dfrac{9}{12}$ f. $\dfrac{16}{20}$

ANSWERS

1 **Addition**

    a. 12   b. 15   c. 16

    d. 10   e. 11   f. 9

2 **Addition**

    a. 0.9   b. 1.2   c. 1.1

    d. 1.4   e. 1.5   f. 0.8

3 **Subtraction**

    a. 4   b. 1   c. 3

    d. 2   e. 3   f. 4

4 **Subtraction**

    a. 0.2   b. 0.1   c. 0.5

    d. 0.2   e. 0.7   f. 0.2

5 **Multiplication**

    a. 40   b. 60   c. 80

    d. 50   e. 70   f. 90

6 **Multiplication**

    a. 5   b. 7   c. 4

    d. 8   e. 3   f. 1

7 **Multiplication**

    a. 20   b. 18   c. 32

    d. 35   e. 24   f. 18

8 **Multiplication**

    a. 112   b. 44   c. 84

    d. 51   e. 90   f. 65

9 **Division**

    a. 0.3   b. 0.8   c. 0.5

    d. 0.4   e. 0.9   f. 0.6

10 **Division**

    a. 0.62   b. 0.98   c. 0.79

    d. 0.55   e. 0.41   f. 0.87

11 **Division**

    a. 4   b. 2   c. 3

    d. 5   c. 2   f. 2

12 **Division**

    a. 7   b. 6   c. 5

    d. 3   e. 14   f. 7

13 **Simplification**

    a. $\dfrac{2}{1}$ b. $\dfrac{2}{1}$ c. $\dfrac{3}{2}$

    d. $\dfrac{1}{3}$ e. $\dfrac{1}{3}$ f. $\dfrac{1}{6}$

14 **Simplification**

    a. $\dfrac{7}{1}$ b. $\dfrac{6}{1}$ c. $\dfrac{8}{1}$

    d. $\dfrac{1}{12}$ e. $\dfrac{2}{3}$ f. $\dfrac{1}{3}$

15 **Simplification**

a. $\dfrac{4}{5}$
b. $\dfrac{7}{9}$
c. $\dfrac{8}{15}$

d. $\dfrac{6}{5}$
e. $\dfrac{7}{6}$
f. $\dfrac{7}{6}$

16 **Simplification**

a. $\dfrac{2}{1}$
b. $\dfrac{2}{1}$
c. $\dfrac{2}{1}$

d. $\dfrac{1}{2}$
e. $\dfrac{2}{1}$
f. $\dfrac{3}{1}$

17 **Round to one decimal place**

a. 0.5
b. 0.9
c. 0.9

d. 1.2
e. 3.8
f. 4.6

18 **Round to two decimal places**

a. 5.88
b. 9.00
c. 6.33

d. 5.23
e. 3.76
f. 2.50

19 **Round to three decimal places**

a. 1.017
b. 3.683
c. 7.555

d. 6.434
e. 4.833
f. 5.556

20 **Change to improper fractions**

a. $\dfrac{14}{5}$
b. $\dfrac{31}{8}$
c. $\dfrac{23}{4}$

d. $\dfrac{29}{3}$
e. $\dfrac{79}{9}$
f. $\dfrac{25}{4}$

21 **Change to improper fractions**

a. $\dfrac{137}{14}$ b. $\dfrac{99}{13}$ c. $\dfrac{74}{16}$

d. $\dfrac{170}{27}$ e. $\dfrac{211}{41}$ f. $\dfrac{240}{29}$

22 **Change to mixed numbers**

a. $2\dfrac{3}{4}$ b. $2\dfrac{2}{7}$ c. $4\dfrac{3}{6}$

d. $2\dfrac{3}{5}$ e. $2\dfrac{3}{8}$ f. $4\dfrac{2}{3}$

23 **Change to decimal equivalents**

a. 0.375   b. 0.8   c. 0.25

d. 0.5   e. 0.75   f. 0.75

24 **Change to decimal equivalents**

a. 0.9   b. 0.5   c. 0.25

d. 0.2   e. 0.25   f. 0.125

25 **Convert the following volumes**

a. 0.25 millilitres

b. 0.5 millilitres

c. 0.635 millilitres

d. 1270 microlitres

e. 2630 microlitres

f. 4610 microlitres

26 **Convert the following volumes**

a. 0.1 litres

b. 0.24 litres

c. 0.825 litres

d. 500 millilitres

e. 640 millilitres

f. 785 millilitres

27 **Convert the following weights**
- a. 0.2 grams
- b. 0.375 grams
- c. 0.950 grams
- d. 400 milligrams
- e. 550 milligrams
- f. 684 milligrams

28 **Convert the following weights**
- a. 0.12 kilograms
- b. 0.25 kilograms
- c. 0.588 kilograms
- d. 200 grams
- e. 450 grams
- f. 825 grams

29 **Express as a percentage**

a. 25%	b. 45%	c. 95%
d. 27%	e. 63%	f. 47%

30 **Express as a percentage**

a. 50%	b. 75%	c. 50%
d. 90%	e. 75%	f. 80%

For more information, and instruction on how to solve specific types of calculation, see the relevant chapter.

1 Addition

Addition is the process of adding or combining numbers to find their *sum*. It is signified by the plus sign (+). It is also one of the commonest types of calculation that we routinely carry out. Generally addition gives little cause for concern, as it is constantly used in everyday situations.

In clinical situations addition is used to determine the total number of tablets administered to a patient or to calculate total fluid output over a given period of time.

Addition follows several important patterns. It is *commutative*, which means that when two numbers are added, the order in which they are added does not matter. It is also *associative*, which means that when more than two numbers are added, the order in which they are added does not matter. Repeated addition of 1 (that is, $1 + 1 + 1 + ...$) is the same as counting. Addition of 0 to a number does not change it.

WORKED EXAMPLES: ADDITION

Calculate the following:

$$27.4 + 18$$

STEP 1

Write the numbers to be added in two horizontal lines, below each other, aligning the decimal points. If a number is a whole number (that is, containing no decimal fraction), add a decimal point to the end of the number. Add zeros to empty spaces on the right to line up the columns.

$$\begin{array}{r} 27.4 \\ + 18.0 \\ \hline \end{array}$$

STEP 2

Starting on the right, add the digits in that column and put the answer directly under the column. If the answer is greater than 10, place the last digit under the column and any remaining digits in the column directly to the left (this is commonly referred to as *carry over*).

Add all columns in the same way, being careful to include any digits that have carried over from the previous column.

$$
\begin{array}{r}
2\ 7.4 \\
+\ 1_{1}8.0 \\
\hline
4\ 5\ 4
\end{array}
$$

STEP 3

Place a decimal point in the answer, directly below the decimal point in the number above.

$$
\begin{array}{r}
2\ 7.4 \\
+\ 1_{1}8.0 \\
\hline
4\ 5.4
\end{array}
$$

The answer is **45.4**

We use the same basic procedure for adding larger numbers. Here's how it's done.

Calculate the following:

587.6 + 327.8

STEP 1

Again, write the numbers to be added in two horizontal lines below each other, aligning the decimal points.

$$
\begin{array}{r}
587.6 \\
+\ 327.8
\end{array}
$$

STEP 2

Starting on the right, add the digits in that column, and put the answer directly under the column. Remember, if the answer is greater than 10, place the last digit under the column, and any remaining digits in the column directly to the left.

Add all columns in the same way as above, being careful to include any digits carried over from the previous column.

$$
\begin{array}{r}
5\ 8\ 7\ .6 \\
+\ 3_12_17_1.8 \\
\hline
9\ 1\ 5\ .4
\end{array}
$$

STEP 3

Place a decimal point in the answer, directly below the decimal point in the number above.

$$
\begin{array}{r}
5\ 8\ 7\ .6 \\
+\ 3_12_17_1.8 \\
\hline
9\ 1\ 5\ .4
\end{array}
$$

The answer is **915.4**

To add more than two numbers, we follow these same three steps.

Calculate the following:

12.8 + 27.3 + 16.5 + 24.8

STEP 1

This time write the numbers to be added in four horizontal lines, below each other, again aligning the decimal points.

$$
\begin{array}{r}
12.8 \\
27.3 \\
16.5 \\
+\ 24.8 \\
\hline
\end{array}
$$

STEP 2

Starting on the right, add the digits in that column and put the answer directly under the column. Again, if the answer is greater than 10 (and this is more likely, the greater the size of the column), place the last digit under the column and any remaining digits in the column directly to the left.

Add all columns in the same way as above, being careful to remember any digits carried over from the previous column.

$$
\begin{array}{r}
1\ 2\ .8 \\
2\ 7\ .3 \\
1\ 6\ .5 \\
+\ 2_2 4_2 .8 \\
\hline
8\ 1\ .4
\end{array}
$$

STEP 3

Place a decimal point in the answer, directly below the decimal point in the numbers above.

$$
\begin{array}{r}
1\ 2\ .8 \\
2\ 7\ .3 \\
1\ 6\ .5 \\
+\ 2_2 4_2 .8 \\
\hline
8\ 1\ .4
\end{array}
$$

The answer is   **81.4**

CHECK-UP TEST: ADDITION

Calculate the following:

a. 5 + 6.3

b. 8.7 + 9.7

c. 24.6 + 32.8 + 27.5

d. 53.2 + 36.5 + 61.1

e. 452.4 + 374.6 + 321.8

f. 211.7 + 631.6 + 126.5

ANSWERS

d. 150.8 e. 1148.8 f. 969.8

a. 11.3 b. 18.4 c. 84.9

2 Subtraction

Subtraction involves taking one number away from another to find the *difference* between them. Unlike addition, the order in which numbers are subtracted within a calculation is important. The process is denoted by the minus sign (−). Repeated subtraction of 1 is the same as counting down; subtraction of 0 does not change a number.

In clinical practice, subtraction is used to calculate the difference between fluid input and output, or to work out how long an infusion has been running.

WORKED EXAMPLES: SUBTRACTION

Calculate the following:

$$31.6 - 18.4$$

STEP 1

Write the number to be subtracted directly below the number that it has to be subtracted from. Remember to align the decimal points. If one of the numbers is a whole number – that is, contains no decimal fraction – add a decimal point to the end of it. Add zeros to empty spaces on the right to line up the columns.

$$
\begin{array}{r}
31.6 \\
- 18.4 \\
\hline
\end{array}
$$

STEP 2

Subtract each column, starting on the right and working left. If the digit being subtracted in a column is larger than the digit above it, 'borrow' a digit from the next column to the left. If you are required to do this, make sure you 'pay back' the 'borrowed' digit.

$$
\begin{array}{r}
3\ 1^1.6 \\
-\ 1_18\ .4 \\
\hline
1\ 3\ \ 2
\end{array}
$$

STEP 3

Place the decimal point in the answer directly below the decimal points in the numbers above.

$$
\begin{array}{r}
3\ 1^1.6 \\
-\ 1_18\ .4 \\
\hline
1\ 3\ \ 2
\end{array}
$$

The answer is   **13.2**

STEP 4

Check your answer by adding the result to the number you subtracted. The sum should equal the number you started with.

$$
\begin{array}{r}
1\ \ 3.2 \\
+\ 1_18.4 \\
\hline
3\ \ 1.6
\end{array}
$$

For larger numbers the same rules apply as above. Here's how it's done.
Calculate the following:

594.2 – 318.6

STEP 1

Write the number to be subtracted directly below the number that it has to be subtracted from. Remember to align the decimal points. If any of the numbers is a whole number – that is, contains no decimal fraction – add a decimal point to the end of it. Add zeros to empty spaces on the right to line up the columns.

$$
\begin{array}{r}
594.2 \\
-\ 318.6 \\
\end{array}
$$

STEP 2

Subtract each column, starting on the right and working left. Again, if the digit being subtracted in a column is larger than the digit above it, 'borrow' a digit from the next column to the left. Remember to 'pay back' the digit that has been 'borrowed'.

$$
\begin{array}{r}
59^{1}4\ .^{1}2 \\
-\ 31_{1}8_{1}.\ 6 \\
\hline
27\ 5\quad 6 \\
\end{array}
$$

STEP 3

Place the decimal point in the answer directly below the decimal points in the numbers above.

$$
\begin{array}{r}
59^{1}4\ .^{1}2 \\
-\ 31_{1}8_{1}.\ 6 \\
\hline
27\ 5\quad 6 \\
\end{array}
$$

The answer is **275.6**

STEP 4

Check your answer by adding the result to the number you subtracted. The sum should equal the number you started with.

$$
\begin{array}{r}
27\ 5\ .6 \\
+\ 31_{1}8_{1}.6 \\
\hline
59\ 4\ .2 \\
\end{array}
$$

CHECK-UP TEST: SUBTRACTION

Calculate the following:

a. 9 – 4.7

b. 9.7 – 4.8

c. 27.3 – 16.4

d. 43.5 – 36.9

e. 412.4 – 361.6

f. 636.1 – 482.6

ANSWERS

f. 153.5   e. 50.8   d. 6.6

c. 10.9   b. 4.9   a. 4.3

3 | Multiplication

Multiplication can be thought of as repeated addition. A number is added to itself a specific number of times, forming a *product*. The numbers that are multiplied to form the product are termed *factors*. Multiplication is represented by the symbol ×. Multiplying any number by 1 does not change it; multiplying any number by 0 always results in a product (or answer) that equals 0.

In clinical practice, multiplication is used to calculate the number of tablets a patient should receive for a prescribed dose, or to estimate certain physiological events, such as heart rate.

WORKED EXAMPLES: MULTIPLICATION

Calculate the following:

82 × 5.3

STEP 1

Write the numbers to be multiplied in two horizontal lines, one below the other, aligning any decimal points.

$$\begin{array}{r} 82 \\ \times\,5.3 \\ \hline \end{array}$$

STEP 2

Start from the right and multiply the numbers 3 × 2 = 6, then multiply the numbers 3 × 8 = 24. Write this down from left to right as 246, as shown below. Place 246 below the drawn line. Make sure that each digit is correctly lined up, as shown below. This is the first line.

$$82$$
$$\times 5.3$$
$$\overline{24\ 6} \quad \text{line 1}$$

STEP 3

Start from the right again and write down 0 as a place holder in the end digit column (this helps line up the relevant digits); then multiply $5 \times 2 = 10$. Write down 0 and carry the 1 over, then multiply $5 \times 8 = 40$ and add the carried-over 1, so $40 + 1 = 41$. Again, write this down from left to right, to give 4100. This is the second line.

$$82$$
$$\times 5.3$$
$$\overline{24\ 6} \quad \text{line 1}$$
$$410\ 0 \quad \text{line 2}$$

STEP 4

Add line 1 and line 2 to get $246 + 4100 = 4346$, and count the number of digits after the decimal points in both factors. In this case there is only one decimal point, with one digit after it, and this needs to be accounted for in the final answer. Insert the decimal point one place from the right to give the correct answer.

$$82$$
$$\times 5.3$$
$$\overline{24\ 6} \quad \text{line 1}$$
$$\underline{410\ 0} \quad \text{line 2}$$
$$434\ 6$$

The answer is **434.6**

The same rules apply when multiplying larger numbers. The only difference is that you must remember to include additional place holders. Here's how it's done.

Calculate the following:

5769 × 7.4

STEP 1

Write the numbers to be multiplied in two horizontal lines, below each other, aligning any decimal points.

$$5769$$
$$\times \quad 7.4$$

STEP 2

Start from the right and multiply the digits 4 × 9 = 36. At the far right, write down the 6 then carry over 3. Then multiply 4 × 6 = 24 and add the carried-over 3 to give 27. To the left of the 6, write down 7 and carry over the 2. Multiply 4 × 7 = 28 and add the carried-over 2 to give 30. To the left of the 7, write down 0 and carry over the 3. Finally, multiply 4 × 5 = 20 and add the carried-over 3 to give 23. Write this 23 down to the left of the 0 to give the final number, 23076. This is the first line.

$$5769$$
$$\times \quad 7.4$$
$$2307\ 6 \quad \text{line 1}$$

STEP 3

Start from the right again, and write down 0 as a place holder in the end digit column; then multiply 7 × 9 = 63. Write down 3 and carry the 6 over; then multiply 7 × 6 = 42 and add the carried-over 6, so 42 + 6 = 48. Again, write 8 down on the left of the 3 and carry over the 4. Multiply 7 × 7 = 49 and add the carried-over 4, giving 53. Write the 3 on the left of the 5 and carry over the 5. Finally, multiply 7 × 5 = 35 and add the carried-over 5 to give 40. Write this down to the left of the 3. Reading from left to right gives the number 403830. This is the second line.

```
        5769
    ×    7.4
     2307 6    line 1
    40383 0    line 2
```

STEP 4

Add line 1 and line 2 to get 23076 + 403830 = 426906, and count the number of digits after the decimal points in both factors. In this case there is one decimal point, with one digit after it, and this needs to be accounted for in the final answer. Insert the decimal point one place from the right to give the correct answer.

```
        5769
    ×    7.4
     2307 6    line 1
    40383 0    line 2
    42690.6
```

The answer is **42690.6**

When multiplying two numbers that both contain decimal fractions, we apply the same rules. Here's how it's done.
Calculate the following:

13.7 × 4.6

STEP 1

Write the numbers to be multiplied in two horizontal lines below each other, aligning any decimal points.

```
    13.7
   ×4.6
```

STEP 2

Start from the right and multiply the numbers 6 × 7 = 42. At the far right, write down 2 and carry over the 4. Then multiply 6 × 3 = 18 and add the carried-over 4 to give 22. To the left of the 2, write down 2 and carry over the remaining 2. Multiply 6 × 1 = 6 and add the carried-over 2 to give 8. Write down 8 to the left of the 2. This gives the number 822 and is the first line.

$$
\begin{array}{r}
13.7 \\
\times 4.6 \\
\hline
82\ 2 \quad \text{line 1}
\end{array}
$$

STEP 3

Start from the right again and write down 0 as a place holder in the end digit column; then multiply 4 × 7 = 28. Write down 8 and carry the 2 over; then multiply 4 × 3 = 12 and add the carried-over 2 to give 14. Write down the 4 to the left of the 8, and carry over the 1. Finally, multiply 4 × 1 and add the carried-over 1 to give 5. Write this down to the left of the 4. This gives the number 5480 and is the second line.

$$
\begin{array}{r}
13.7 \\
\times 4.6 \\
\hline
82\ 2 \quad \text{line 1} \\
548\ 0 \quad \text{line 2}
\end{array}
$$

STEP 4

Add line 1 and line 2 to get 822 + 5480 = 6302 and count the number of digits after the decimal points in both factors.

In this case there are two decimal fractions, each with one digit after it, which need to be accounted for in the final answer. Insert the decimal point two places from the right to give the correct answer.

```
       13.7
      ×4.6
      82 2    line 1
      548 0   line 2
      63.02
```

The answer is   **63.02**

 CHECK-UP TEST: MULTIPLICATION

Calculate the following:

a.   8 × 5.9

b.   5 × 6.8

c.   7 × 81.4

d.   6 × 63.6

e.   4.4 × 361.6

f.   6.5 × 712.5

ANSWERS

d. 381.6   e. 1591.04   f. 4631.25

a. 47.2   b. 34   c. 569.8

4 Division

Division is the process of separating a number into a specified number of equal parts. The result is known as the *quotient*. The number that is divided is called the *dividend,* and the number that divides it is called the *divisor*. Division is represented by the ÷ symbol. Dividing any number by 1 does not change the number.

In clinical practice, division is used to calculate the number of tablets or amount of a drug to be given in divided doses, or the frequency with which a physiological event occurs over a period of time.

WORKED EXAMPLES: DIVISION

Calculate the following:

$$25 \div 5$$

STEP 1

Understand the terms. The dividend is the number that is divided, or the number under the division bracket when we write the calculation out (see below). The divisor is the number that does the dividing.

In this example 25 is the dividend, and 5 is the divisor. We can write the calculation as:

$$5 \overline{)25}$$

STEP 2

Divide the dividend by the divisor to reach the answer.

$$5 \overline{)25}^{\,5}$$

The answer is **5**

In this case the dividend is exactly divisible by the divisor, leaving no remainder. The basic process is similar for the division of larger whole numbers. Let's look at another example.

Calculate the following:

378 ÷ 8

STEP 1

Understand the terms. The dividend is the number that is divided, or the number under the division bracket when we write the calculation out. The divisor is the number that does the dividing.

In this example 378 is the dividend, and 8 is the divisor.

$$8 \overline{)3\ 7\ 8}$$

STEP 2

Divide the dividend by the divisor to reach the answer. In this case 8 will not divide into 3, but will divide 4 times into 37, giving 32 with a remainder of 5. Place the 4 on the top of the dividing bracket in line with the 7 of the dividend. The 32 is written below the 3 and 7 of the dividend.

Using subtraction, 37 minus 32 equals 5 (which represents the remainder). This is written below the digit 2 of '32'. As the number 5 can not be divided by 8, we need to bring down the 8 from the dividend, to give 58. This number can be divided 7 times by 8, giving 56 with a remainder of 2. The 7 is written above the dividing bracket, to the right of the 4. The 56 is written below the 58. Again, using subtraction, 58 minus 56 equals 2 (which is the remainder) and is placed under the 6 of the 56.

This remaining 2 is not divisible by 8, so we need to insert a decimal point after the 378 under the bracket and a zero is brought down to make 20. This 20 can be divided twice by 8, giving 16 and leaving a remainder of 4. The 2 is written above the bracket to the right of the decimal point. The 16 is written below the 20. Again using subtraction, 20 minus 16 equals 4 (the remainder).

Another zero must be brought down as the 4 is not divisible by 8. This gives 40 which is exactly divisible by 8 giving 5, with no remainder. Write the 5 above the bracket to the right of the 2. Place the decimal point in the answer directly above the decimal point in the dividend below the bracket.

$$\begin{array}{r} 47.25 \\ 8\overline{)378.00} \\ 32 \\ \hline 58 \\ -56 \\ \hline 20 \\ -16 \\ \hline 40 \\ -40 \\ \hline 0 \end{array}$$

The answer is **47.25**

If the divisor is not a whole number, move the decimal point to right to make it a whole number, and move the decimal point in the dividend to the right by the same number of places, as shown in the example below.

Calculate the following:

97.68 ÷ 3.7

STEP 1

Understand the terms. The dividend is the number that is divided, or the number under the division bracket when we write the calculation out. The divisor is the number that does the dividing.

In this example, 97.68 is the dividend and 3.7 is the divisor.

$$3.7\overline{)97.68}$$

STEP 2

Move the decimal point in the divisor one place to the right to make it a whole number, and move the decimal point in the dividend the same number of places.

$$37\overline{)976.8}$$

STEP 3

Divide as usual. Keep dividing until the answer terminates, as it did in the previous example, or repeats (sometimes it's not possible to reach an exact answer, and the final digits keep repeating, or *recurring*). Put the decimal point in the answer directly above the decimal point in the dividend.

$$
\begin{array}{r}
2\,6\,.4 \\
37\,\overline{)\,9\,7\,6\,.8} \\
-\,7\,4 \\
\hline
2\,3\,6 \\
-\,2\,2\,2 \\
\hline
1\,4\,8 \\
-\,1\,4\,8 \\
\hline
0
\end{array}
$$

The answer is **26.4**

STEP 4

To check your answer, multiply the quotient by the divisor. To see how best to do this remember to check the previous chapter.

$$
\begin{array}{r}
2\,6\,.4 \\
\times\,3\,7 \\
\hline
9\,7\,6\,.8
\end{array}
$$

CHECK-UP TEST: DIVISION

Calculate the following:

a. 88 ÷ 4

b. 72 ÷ 8

c. 20 ÷ 2.5

d. 128 ÷ 25.6

e. 537.5 ÷ 4.3

f. 183.6 ÷ 15.3

ANSWERS

d. 5   e. 125   f. 12

a. 22   b. 9   c. 8

5 Simplification

Simplification involves cancelling down fractions, and requires an understanding of *factors* (see Chapter 3 on multiplication). When we divide a number by one of its factors, the answer is a whole number.

To simplify a fraction, divide the *numerator* (the top number) and the *denominator* (the bottom number) by the same amount. Fractions are easier to manipulate if they are reduced to their lowest denominator.

When comparing the size of different fractions it is useful to determine the *lowest common denominator*. There is no definitive method for identifying the lowest common denominator, and it is often a matter of trial and error. However, there are some useful number patterns that help make calculations involving fractions a lot easier. For instance, even numbers (2, 4, 6, . . .) can always be divided by 2, and sometimes by multiples of 2. Numbers ending in 5 or 0 can always be divided by 5.

WORKED EXAMPLES: SIMPLIFICATION

Simplify the following fraction:

$$\frac{84}{126}$$

STEP 1

Identify the common factors of the numerator and denominator, by listing the numbers that divide into both of them to give a whole number.
The factors of the numerator, 84, are:

$$1, 2, 3, 4, 6, 7, 12, 14, 21, 28, 42, 84$$

The factors of the denominator, 126, are:

$$1, 2, 3, 6, 7, 9, 14, 18, 21, 42, 63, 126$$

The common factors are therefore:

$$1, 2, 3, 6, 7, 14, 21, 42$$

STEP 2

Divide both the numerator and denominator by the highest common factor, which in this case is 42.

$$\frac{\cancel{84}^{2}}{\cancel{126}_{3}} = \frac{2}{3}$$

The answer is $\dfrac{2}{3}$

The same basic principles apply to situations that require fractions to be compared.

Arrange the following fractions in order of increasing size:

$$\frac{4}{5} \quad \frac{2}{3} \quad \frac{3}{4}$$

STEP 1

This part involves trial and error. First, we need to express all three fractions in terms of the same denominator (the *common denominator*). The simplest way to do this is to multiply the three denominators together.

$$5 \times 3 \times 4 = 60$$

Now, to make the numbers more manageable, look to see whether there is a smaller number that each of the three original denominators will divide into (the *lowest common denominator*). In this case, though, the smallest number that each of these denominators will divide into is 60, so no reduction in the common denominator is possible.

STEP 2

For each fraction, multiply the numerator by the denominators of the other two fractions, so that all three have the same (common) denominator. Multiply the numerator of the fraction by the same number as the denominator, so that the overall size of the fraction is not changed.

To change $\frac{4}{5}$ multiply both the numerator and denominator by $3 \times 4 = 12$.

This gives $\frac{48}{60}$.

To change $\frac{2}{3}$ multiply both the numerator and the denominator by $5 \times 4 = 20$.

This gives $\frac{40}{60}$.

To change $\frac{3}{4}$ multiply both the numerator and the denominator by $5 \times 3 = 15$.

This gives $\frac{45}{60}$.

STEP 3

Rearrange these in increasing size, and then convert back to the original fractions.

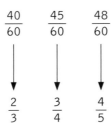

$$\frac{40}{60} \qquad \frac{45}{60} \qquad \frac{48}{60}$$

$$\frac{2}{3} \qquad \frac{3}{4} \qquad \frac{4}{5}$$

CHECK-UP TEST: SIMPLIFICATION

Simplify the following:

a. $\dfrac{7}{21}$

b. $\dfrac{16}{20}$

c. $\dfrac{121}{132}$

Arrange the following fractions in order of increasing size:

d. $\dfrac{8}{11}$ $\dfrac{7}{12}$ $\dfrac{3}{4}$

e. $\dfrac{4}{7}$ $\dfrac{8}{9}$ $\dfrac{18}{21}$

f. $\dfrac{1}{2}$ $\dfrac{7}{8}$ $\dfrac{3}{4}$

ANSWERS

d. $\dfrac{12}{7}$ $\dfrac{11}{8}$ $\dfrac{4}{3}$ e. $\dfrac{7}{4}$ $\dfrac{21}{18}$ $\dfrac{9}{8}$ f. $\dfrac{1}{2}$ $\dfrac{3}{4}$ $\dfrac{8}{7}$

a. $\dfrac{1}{3}$ b. $\dfrac{4}{5}$ c. $\dfrac{11}{12}$

6 Rounding

When you are calculating with decimal fractions, many of the small decimals may become irrelevant, because they are so small in relation to the size of the overall number. In this situation you need to *round* numbers with long decimal fractions, to reduce the number of decimal places. Here's how it's done.

First, determine the number of decimal places to the right of the decimal point that you need. Then, if the digit to the right of the last of these decimal places is 4 or less, it is irrelevant, and you can ignore it. If it is 5 or more, then add 1 to the digit to the left and delete the irrelevant digits to the right.

In clinical situations it can be useful to round numbers when dealing with weights or volumes that have a large number of decimal places. The amount of rounding needed depends on the particular situation.

WORKED EXAMPLES: ROUNDING

Round the following decimal fraction to two decimal places:

8.3379

STEP 1

Separate the number between the relevant decimal places – in this case, between the second and third decimal places.

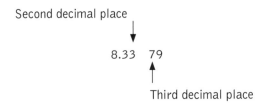

Second decimal place

8.33 79

Third decimal place

STEP 2

Look at the third decimal place. In this case, 7 is greater than 5, so add 1 to the digit on the left.

8.33   79

+ 1

STEP 3

Delete the irrelevant digits to the right.

8.34

The answer is **8.34**

The same basic principles apply to numbers that require rounding down.
Round the following decimal fraction to three decimal places:

7.54342

STEP 1

Separate the number between the relevant decimal places – in this case, between the third and fourth decimal places.

Third decimal place

7.543   42

Fourth decimal place

STEP 2

Look at the fourth decimal place. In this case 4 is less than 5, and so the 3 remains. Rounding is not required.

7.543   42

STEP 3

Delete the irrelevant digits to the right.

7.543

The answer is **7.543**

CHECK-UP TEST: ROUNDING

Round the following numbers to the specified number of decimal places:

a.   4.2567   to 3 decimal places

b.   8.2723   to 2 decimal places

c.   16.455   to 1 decimal place

d.   12.437   to 2 decimal places

e.   8.994   to 2 decimal places

f.   4.995   to 2 decimal places

ANSWERS

d. 12.44   e. 8.99   f. 5.00

a. 4.257   b. 8.27   c. 16.5

7 Improper fractions

Improper fractions are fractions in which the *numerator* (the top number) is greater than the *denominator* (the bottom number). They are commonly used in number calculations. An improper fraction can also be expressed as a *mixed number* – a number that contains both a whole number and a fraction. It is generally easier to work with improper fractions than with mixed numbers.

Converting mixed numbers to improper fractions is a reasonably straightforward process.

WORKED EXAMPLE: IMPROPER FRACTIONS

Convert the following mixed number to an improper fraction:

$$12\frac{5}{9}$$

STEP 1

Multiply the denominator of the fraction by the whole number.

$$12 \times 9 = 108$$

STEP 2

Add the resulting number from step 1 to the numerator of the fraction to form a new numerator.

$$108 + 5 = 113$$

STEP 3

Leave the denominator as it is.

$$12\frac{5}{9} = \frac{113}{9}$$

The answer is $\dfrac{113}{9}$

 CHECK-UP TEST: IMPROPER FRACTIONS

Change the following mixed numbers to improper fractions:

a. $4\frac{8}{9}$

b. $9\frac{6}{8}$

c. $16\frac{11}{20}$

d. $24\frac{21}{25}$

e. $34\frac{26}{42}$

f. $41\frac{43}{47}$

ANSWERS

d. $\dfrac{621}{25}$ e. $\dfrac{1454}{42}$ f. $\dfrac{1970}{47}$

a. $\dfrac{44}{9}$ b. $\dfrac{78}{8}$ c. $\dfrac{331}{20}$

8 Mixed numbers

Mixed numbers can be considered as an alternative way of presenting improper fractions. When comparing improper fractions it is often useful to convert them to mixed numbers. The process is essentially the opposite of that shown in Chapter 7.

WORKED EXAMPLE: MIXED NUMBERS

Convert the following improper fraction to a mixed number:

$$\frac{11}{3}$$

STEP 1

Divide the numerator (top number) by the denominator (bottom number). In this case we get 3 (which becomes the whole number), with a remainder of 2.

$$\frac{11}{3} = 3 \text{ remainder } 2$$

STEP 2

The remainder becomes the new numerator in the fraction, and the denominator remains the same.

$$\frac{11}{3} = 3\frac{2}{3}$$

The answer is $\mathbf{3\frac{2}{3}}$

CHECK-UP TEST: MIXED NUMBERS

Change the following improper fractions to mixed numbers:

a. $\dfrac{8}{5}$

b. $\dfrac{5}{3}$

c. $\dfrac{13}{6}$

d. $\dfrac{21}{5}$

e. $\dfrac{231}{36}$

f. $\dfrac{311}{42}$

ANSWERS

d. $4\dfrac{1}{5}$

e. $6\dfrac{15}{36}$

f. $7\dfrac{17}{42}$

a. $1\dfrac{3}{5}$

b. $1\dfrac{2}{3}$

c. $2\dfrac{1}{6}$

9 Decimal conversions

Decimals are a way of writing fractions without using a numerator or a denominator. Instead, we use a decimal point to distinguish between whole numbers and fractions. Whole numbers appear to the left of the decimal point, and decimal fractions to the right. The value of an individual digit within a decimal depends on its position in the number. Each place to the left of the decimal point is greater than the previous one by a magnitude of 10. Each place to the right of the decimal point is smaller than the previous one by a factor of 10.

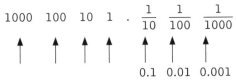

$$1000 \quad 100 \quad 10 \quad 1 \quad . \quad \frac{1}{10} \quad \frac{1}{100} \quad \frac{1}{1000}$$

$$0.1 \quad 0.01 \quad 0.001$$

In many ways, decimal fractions are easier to work with than conventional fractions although sometimes you may need to convert between the two. This chapter will show you how.

We have covered the basic functions of addition, subtraction, multiplication and division of decimals in previous chapters.

WORKED EXAMPLES: DECIMAL CONVERSIONS

Convert the following decimal to a fraction:

14.231

STEP 1

To convert a decimal to a fraction, count the number of decimal places the decimal has. For the denominator (bottom line) of the fraction, put a 1 followed by as many zeros as there are decimal places. If you have 2 decimal places, the denominator would be 100. If you have 4 decimal places, the denominator would be 10000.

We can therefore represent the number 14.231 as 14 and 231 thousandths.

STEP 2

Count the number of places to the right of the decimal point. This equates to the number of zeros in the denominator of the fraction.

$$14.231 = 14\,\frac{231}{1000}$$

The answer is $14\dfrac{231}{1000}$

To *convert fractions to decimals,* divide the numerator by the denominator. Place the decimal point to the right of the numerator, and add zeros after the decimal point to help with the calculation. Determine the number of decimal places that are required in the answer, and round off as needed. If the fraction is a mixed number, convert it to an improper fraction before proceeding.

Convert the following fraction to a decimal number:

$4\dfrac{5}{8}$

STEP 1

Since this is a mixed number it must be converted to an improper fraction. Multiply the denominator (the bottom line) by the whole number.

$$4 \times 8 = 32$$

STEP 2

Add the resulting number from step 1 to the numerator to form a new numerator.

$$32 + 5 = 37$$

STEP 3

Leave the denominator as it is.

$$4\frac{5}{8} = \frac{37}{8}$$

STEP 4

Place the decimal point to the right of the numerator and add zeros to help with the calculation.

$$8\overline{)37.000}$$

STEP 5

Keep dividing until the answer terminates or repeats. Put the decimal point directly above the decimal point in the dividend.

$$
\begin{array}{r}
4.625 \\
8\overline{)37.000} \\
-\underline{32} \\
50 \\
-\underline{48} \\
20 \\
-\underline{16} \\
40 \\
-\underline{40} \\
0
\end{array}
$$

The answer is **4.625**

CHECK-UP TEST: DECIMAL CONVERSIONS

Convert the following decimals to fractions:

a. 11.2

b. 114.75

c. 650.452

Convert the following fractions to decimals:

d. $6\frac{1}{4}$

e. $114\frac{16}{20}$

f. $823\frac{562}{1000}$

ANSWERS

d. 6.25   e. 114.8   f. 823.562

a. $11\frac{2}{10}$ b. $114\frac{75}{100}$ c. $650\frac{452}{1000}$

10 Unit conversions

The metric system of measurement relies on decimals. It is a useful system, because it eliminates common fractions, simplifies the calculation of large and small units of measurement, and has been adopted by most countries of the world.

The basic units of measurement in this system are the metre (length [m]), litre (volume [L]) and kilogram (weight [kg]).

Multiples and subdivisions of these units are indicated by a prefix before the basic unit, and each prefix used in the system represents a multiple of 10, as listed in Table 1.

Table 1: Common metric prefixes

Prefix	Symbol	Multiple of 10	
kilo	k	1000	
hecto	h	100	
deca	da	10	
deci	d	0.1	(1/10)
centi	c	0.01	(1/100)
milli	m	0.001	(1/1000)
micro	mc	0.000001	(1/1000000)

Since the metric system is based on decimals, it is fairly easy to convert from one metric unit to another.

To convert a smaller unit to a larger unit, we move the decimal point to the left.

To convert a larger unit to a smaller unit, we move the decimal point to the right.

WORKED EXAMPLES: UNIT CONVERSIONS

Convert the following:

1.7 metres to centimetres

STEP 1

Understand the prefixes, as shown in Table 1. From the table you can see that the prefix *centi* refers to hundredths: in this example we are talking about hundredths of a metre.

STEP 2

Multiply the number of metres by 100, because we are converting from metres to centimetres.

$$1.7 \times 100 = 170$$

STEP 3

Remember to include the units; measurements are meaningless without them. In examinations you will be penalized for answers that do not include the correct units.

$$1.7 \times 100 = 170 \text{ centimetres}$$

The answer is **170 centimetres**

Convert the following:

1.45 litres to millilitres

STEP 1

Again, make sure you understand the prefixes as shown in Table 1. From the table you can see that the prefix *milli* refers to thousandths: in this case we are referring to volume, and to thousandths of a litre.

STEP 2

Multiply the number of litres by 1000.

$$1.45 \times 1000 = 1450$$

STEP 3

Finally, include the relevant units.

$$1.45 \times 1000 = 1450 \text{ millilitres}$$

The answer is **1450 millilitres**

Convert the following:

8400 grams to kilograms

STEP 1

Again, make sure you understand the connections between the prefixes in Table 1. This time we are looking at a reduction in the size of the number, as there are 1000 g in 1 kg. Reduction requires division.

STEP 2

Divide the number of grams by 1000.

$$8400 \div 1000 = 8.4$$

STEP 3

Include the relevant units.

8400 ÷ 1000 = 8.4 kilograms

The answer is **8.4 kilograms**

 CHECK-UP TEST: UNIT CONVERSIONS

Convert the following:

a. 7.6 millilitres to microlitres

b. 4.95 metres to millimetres

c. 2.545 grams to milligrams

d. 225 millilitres to litres

e. 11.54 centimetres to metres

f. 250 micrograms to milligrams

ANSWERS

d. 0.225 litres   e. 0.1154 metres   f. 0.25 milligrams

a. 7600 microlitres   b. 4950 millimetres   c. 2545 milligrams

11 Percentages

A percentage is an alternative way of expressing a fraction, as a proportion of 100. It is represented by the percentage sign (%). If expressed as a fraction, its denominator would be 100. If expressed as a decimal, it would have two decimal places.

To change a decimal to a percentage, move the decimal point two places to the right, and add the percent sign.

WORKED EXAMPLES: PERCENTAGES

Convert the following decimal to a percentage:

0.035

STEP 1

Move the decimal point two places to the right (multiply by 100).

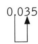

STEP 2

Add the percentage sign.

3.5%

The answer is **3.5%**

To change a percentage to a decimal, remove the percentage sign and move the decimal point two places to the left (divide by 100).
Convert the following percentage to a decimal.

18.4%

STEP 1

Remove the percentage sign.

18.4

STEP 2

Move the decimal point two places to the left.

18.4

STEP 3

Add a zero as a place holder.

0.184

The answer is **0.184**

CHECK-UP TEST: PERCENTAGES

Convert the following decimals to percentages:

a. 0.027

b. 0.85

c. 1.36

Convert the following percentages to decimals:

d. 3.8%

e. 72.4%

f. 212.8%

ANSWERS

d. 0.038   e. 0.724   f. 2.128

a. 2.7%   b. 85%   c. 136%

FOR EACH OF THE FOLLOWING CALCULATE THE CORRECT ANSWER

1 **Addition**

   a. 5 + 9   b. 8 + 7   c. 6 + 8

   d. 9 + 7   e. 5 + 2   f. 9 + 2

2 **Addition**

   a. 0.4 + 0.7   b. 0.6 + 0.9   c. 0.4 + 0.2

   d. 0.3 + 0.9   e. 0.9 + 0.9   f. 0.5 + 0.6

3 **Subtraction**

   a. 8 − 2   b. 9 − 3   c. 9 − 1

   d. 7 − 3   e. 8 − 4   f. 6 − 5

4 **Subtraction**

   a. 0.7 − 0.6   b. 0.9 − 0.3   c. 0.7 − 0.5

   d. 0.9 − 0.4   e. 0.5 − 0.2   f. 0.8 − 0.1

5 | Multiplication

a. 3×10 b. 4×10 c. 5×10

d. 6×10 e. 2×10 f. 8×10

6 | Multiplication

a. 0.2×10 b. 0.9×10 c. 0.5×10

d. 0.7×10 e. 0.4×10 e. 0.6×10

7 | Multiplication

a. 6×3 b. 9×2 c. 7×8

d. 5×3 e. 3×9 f. 4×9

8 | Multiplication

a. 11×7 b. 12×4 c. 16×8

d. 15×3 e. 45×3 f. 12×7

9 | Division

a. $4 \div 10$ b. $7 \div 10$ c. $9 \div 10$

d. $5 \div 10$ e. $3 \div 10$ f. $8 \div 10$

10 | Division

a. $4.7 \div 10$ b. $7.2 \div 10$ c. $6.8 \div 10$

d. $6.9 \div 10$ e. $4.6 \div 10$ f. $5.9 \div 10$

11 **Division**

   a. $9 \div 3$ b. $8 \div 2$ c. $6 \div 3$

   d. $4 \div 4$ e. $7 \div 1$ f. $8 \div 4$

12 **Division**

   a. $15 \div 3$ b. $27 \div 3$ c. $18 \div 2$

   d. $24 \div 8$ e. $26 \div 2$ f. $42 \div 7$

13 **Simplification**

   a. $\dfrac{8}{2}$ b. $\dfrac{9}{3}$ c. $\dfrac{8}{4}$

   d. $\dfrac{2}{8}$ e. $\dfrac{3}{6}$ f. $\dfrac{6}{18}$

14 **Simplification**

   a. $\dfrac{24}{2}$ b. $\dfrac{24}{3}$ c. $\dfrac{56}{7}$

   d. $\dfrac{12}{36}$ e. $\dfrac{15}{45}$ f. $\dfrac{9}{27}$

15 **Simplification**

   a. $\dfrac{410}{500}$ b. $\dfrac{360}{470}$ c. $\dfrac{20}{620}$

   d. $\dfrac{270}{400}$ e. $\dfrac{330}{520}$ f. $\dfrac{300}{680}$

16 **Simplification**

a. $\dfrac{0.6}{0.2}$ b. $\dfrac{0.9}{0.3}$ c. $\dfrac{0.8}{0.2}$

d. $\dfrac{0.2}{0.8}$ e. $\dfrac{0.8}{0.4}$ f. $\dfrac{0.6}{0.3}$

17 **Round to one decimal place**

a. 0.53   b. 0.67   c. 0.56

d. 2.84   e. 5.82   f. 6.65

18 **Round to two decimal places**

a. 6.857   b. 9.295   c. 7.357

d. 9.587   e. 8.455   f. 9.216

19 **Round to three decimal places**

a. 2.7854   b. 7.5645   c. 6.2222

d. 6.5887   e. 8.4332   f. 7.6664

20 **Change to improper fractions**

a. $3\dfrac{3}{5}$ b. $4\dfrac{6}{9}$ c. $8\dfrac{3}{5}$

d. $9\dfrac{2}{9}$ e. $5\dfrac{4}{9}$ f. $5\dfrac{3}{7}$

21 **Change to improper fractions**

a. $5\frac{16}{18}$　　　b. $6\frac{9}{13}$　　　c. $5\frac{7}{16}$

d. $2\frac{11}{27}$　　　e. $4\frac{6}{34}$　　　f. $8\frac{8}{21}$

22 **Change to mixed numbers**

a. $\frac{17}{5}$　　　b. $\frac{17}{7}$　　　c. $\frac{34}{5}$

d. $\frac{11}{9}$　　　e. $\frac{23}{6}$　　　f. $\frac{17}{4}$

23 **Change to decimal equivalents**

a. $\frac{4}{8}$　　　b. $\frac{3}{5}$　　　c. $\frac{1}{8}$

d. $\frac{3}{4}$　　　e. $\frac{3}{6}$　　　f. $\frac{2}{8}$

24 **Change to decimal equivalents**

a. $\frac{18}{24}$　　　b. $\frac{12}{60}$　　　c. $\frac{21}{25}$

d. $\frac{9}{45}$　　　e. $\frac{17}{34}$　　　f. $\frac{11}{44}$

25 **Convert the following volumes**
  a.   275 microlitres to millilitres
  b.   387 microlitres to millilitres
  c.   415 microlitres to millilitres
  d.   3.25 millilitres to microlitres
  e.   4.68 millilitres to microlitres
  f.   5.82 millilitres to microlitres

26 **Convert the following volumes**
  a.   125 millilitres to litres
  b.   340 millilitres to litres
  c.   615 millilitres to litres
  d.   0.3 litres to millilitres
  e.   0.55 litres to millilitres
  f.   0.685 litres to millilitres

27 **Convert the following weights**
  a.   250 milligrams to grams
  b.   500 milligrams to grams
  c.   750 milligrams to grams
  d.   0.3 grams to milligrams
  e.   0.45 grams to milligrams
  f.   0.721 grams to milligrams

28 **Convert the following weights**
  a.   160 grams to kilograms
  b.   450 grams to kilograms
  c.   725 grams to kilograms
  d.   0.1 kilograms to grams
  e.   0.35 kilograms to grams
  f.   0.755 kilograms to grams

29 **Express as a percentage**

    a. 0.37   b. 0.84   c. 0.91

    d. 0.42   e. 0.75   f. 0.90

30 **Express as a percentage**

    a. $\dfrac{1}{4}$ b. $\dfrac{3}{5}$ c. $\dfrac{2}{8}$

    d. $\dfrac{7}{14}$ e. $\dfrac{6}{24}$ f. $\dfrac{12}{20}$

1 **Addition**

a. 14	b. 15	c. 14
d. 16	e. 7	f. 11

2 **Addition**

a. 1.1	b. 1.5	c. 0.6
d. 1.2	e. 1.8	f. 1.1

3 **Subtraction**

a. 6	b. 6	c. 8
d. 4	e. 4	f. 1

4 **Subtraction**

a. 0.1	b. 0.6	c. 0.2
d. 0.5	e. 0.3	f. 0.7

5 **Multiplication**

a. 30	b. 40	c. 50
d. 60	e. 20	f. 80

6 **Multiplication**

a. 2	b. 9	c. 5
d. 7	e. 4	f. 6

7 **Multiplication**

a. 18	b. 18	c. 56
d. 15	e. 27	f. 36

8 **Multiplication**

    a. 77   b. 48   c. 128

    d. 45   e. 135   f. 84

9 **Division**

    a. 0.4   b. 0.7   c. 0.9

    d. 0.5   e. 0.3   f. 0.8

10 **Division**

    a. 0.47   b. 0.72   c. 0.68

    d. 0.69   e. 0.46   f. 0.59

11 **Division**

    a. 3   b. 4   c. 2

    d. 1   e. 7   f. 2

12 **Division**

    a. 5   b. 9   c. 9

    d. 3   e. 13   f. 6

13 **Simplification**

    a. $\dfrac{4}{1}$ b. $\dfrac{3}{1}$ c. $\dfrac{2}{1}$

    d. $\dfrac{1}{4}$ e. $\dfrac{1}{2}$ f. $\dfrac{1}{3}$

14 **Simplification**

    a. $\dfrac{12}{1}$ b. $\dfrac{8}{1}$ c. $\dfrac{8}{1}$

    d. $\dfrac{1}{3}$ e. $\dfrac{1}{3}$ f. $\dfrac{1}{3}$

15 **Simplification**

a. $\dfrac{41}{50}$ b. $\dfrac{36}{47}$ c. $\dfrac{1}{31}$

d. $\dfrac{27}{40}$ e. $\dfrac{33}{52}$ f. $\dfrac{15}{34}$

16 **Simplification**

a. $\dfrac{3}{1}$ b. $\dfrac{3}{1}$ c. $\dfrac{4}{1}$

d. $\dfrac{1}{4}$ e. $\dfrac{2}{1}$ f. $\dfrac{2}{1}$

17 **Round to one decimal place**

a. 0.5   b. 0.7   c. 0.6

d. 2.8   e. 5.8   f. 6.7

18 **Round to two decimal places**

a. 6.86   b. 9.30   c. 7.36

d. 9.59   e. 8.46   f. 9.22

19 **Round to three decimal places**

a. 2.785   b. 7.565   c. 6.222

d. 6.589   e. 8.433   f. 7.666

20 **Change to improper fractions**

a. $\dfrac{18}{5}$ b. $\dfrac{42}{9}$ c. $\dfrac{43}{5}$

d. $\dfrac{83}{9}$ e. $\dfrac{49}{9}$ f. $\dfrac{38}{7}$

21 **Change to improper fractions**

a. $\dfrac{106}{18}$ b. $\dfrac{87}{13}$ c. $\dfrac{87}{16}$

d. $\dfrac{65}{27}$ e. $\dfrac{142}{34}$ f. $\dfrac{176}{21}$

22 **Change to mixed numbers**

a. $3\dfrac{2}{5}$ b. $2\dfrac{3}{7}$ c. $6\dfrac{4}{5}$

d. $1\dfrac{2}{9}$ e. $3\dfrac{5}{6}$ f. $4\dfrac{1}{4}$

23 **Change to decimal equivalents**

a. 0.5   b. 0.6   c. 0.125

d. 0.75   e. 0.5   f. 0.25

24 **Change to decimal equivalents**

a. 0.75   b. 0.2   c. 0.84

d. 0.2   e. 0.5   f. 0.25

25 **Convert the following volumes**

a. 0.275 millilitres

b. 0.387 millilitres

c. 0.415 millilitres

d. 3250 microlitres

e. 4680 microlitres

f. 5820 microlitres

26 **Convert the following volumes**

a. 0.125 litres

b. 0.340 litres

c. 0.615 litres

d. 300 millilitres

e. 550 millilitres

f. 685 millilitres

27 **Convert the following weights**
a. 0.250 grams
b. 0.500 grams
c. 0.750 grams
d. 300 milligrams
e. 450 milligrams
f. 721 milligrams

28 **Convert the following weights**
a. 0.16 kilograms
b. 0.45 kilograms
c. 0.725 kilograms
d. 100 grams
e. 350 grams
f. 755 grams

29 **Express as a percentage**
a. 37%   b. 84%   c. 91%
d. 42%   e. 75%   f. 90%

30 **Express as a percentage**
a. 25%   b. 60%   c. 25%
d. 50%   e. 25%   f. 60%

Applications review

INTRODUCTION

Drugs are administered by nurses and allied health professionals in many routine and emergency situations. The correct administration of these drugs depends on many factors, of which the correct calculation of dose is only one. However, it is the most frequently cited reason for drug-related errors in the UK, and these can have tragic consequences.

The reasons for calculation errors are many and varied, but by adhering to the simple rules relating to the type and route of drug administration, these errors can be markedly reduced.

Key to the safe and confident administration of drugs is applying and manipulating the correct formula for each administration route. These formulae are detailed in the following chapters, and summarized in the appendix. You need to learn them; knowing which formula to use in each application is the first step in helping you administer drugs safely.

By keeping these formulae in mind, and applying the simple steps you have practised in the previous section, you will become more confident in your handling of drug calculations. More importantly, you will become a safe administrator of medicines.

The following diagnostic test examines your knowledge of the application of the various formulae used in calculating drug doses.

FOR EACH OF THE FOLLOWING CALCULATE THE CORRECT ANSWER

1 | **Oral medication**

A patient is prescribed 1 g paracetamol by mouth. Stock is available in 500 mg tablets. How many tablets should be given?

2 | **Oral medication**

A patient is prescribed 250 mg aspirin. Stock available from the pharmacy comes in 500 mg tablets. How many tablets should be administered?

3 | **Oral medication**

Digoxin is prescribed for a patient at a dose of 250 micrograms. Tablets are available in 0.5 mg dose amounts. How many should be given?

4 | **Oral medication**

15 mg of diazepam are prescribed. The stock available comes in 5 mg tablets. How many should be given?

5 | **Oral medication**

A patient is to receive 80 mg of furosemide. 40 mg tablets are available. How many should the patient be given?

6 | **Oral medication**

A patient requires 200 mg verapamil. Tablets are available in 40 mg doses. How many should the patient be given?

7 | Oral medication

A suspension contains penicillin at 125 mg/5 mL. How many milligrams of penicillin are contained in each of the following volumes?

a. 10 mL   b. 15 mL   c. 20 mL

8 | Oral medication

Paracetamol is available as a suspension containing 200 mg/5 mL. How many milligrams of paracetamol are contained in the following volumes?

a. 10 mL   b. 15 mL   c. 25 mL

9 | Oral medication

Erythromycin is available as a suspension containing 250 mg/5 mL. How much of the drug is contained in these volumes?

a. 7.5 mL   b. 10 mL   c. 15 mL

10 | Oral medication

A suspension of phenytoin contains 125 mg of the drug in 5 mL. How much of the drug is contained in each of the following volumes?

a. 2.5 mL   b. 12.5 mL   c. 25 mL

11 | Oral medication

A patient is prescribed penicillin, 500 mg to be given orally. The suspension contains 500 mg/5 mL. How much should be given?

12 | Oral medication

A patient is prescribed 750 mg of penicillin by mouth. A suspension is available that contains 250 mg/5 mL. How much should be given?

13 | Oral medication

Paracetamol suspension 500 mg is to be given to a patient. The stock contains 250 mg in 5 mL. What volume should be given?

14 **Oral medication**

Penicillin 800 mg is prescribed. A solution containing 250 mg/5 mL is available. What volume should be dispensed?

15 **Oral medication**

Furosemide is to be given at a dose of 125 mg. Available stock is 50 mg/2 mL. What volume should be given?

16 **Injections**

Heparin sodium is available at a strength of 1000 units/mL. A patient is prescribed 2500 units. How much should be drawn up for injection?

17 **Injections**

An injection of digoxin 250 micrograms is required. The drug is available in vials containing 1000 micrograms in 2 mL. How much should be drawn up for injection?

18 **Injections**

A patient is to receive an injection of 600 mg phenoxymethylpenicillin. The drug is available in ampoules containing 250 mg/mL. How much is required for injection?

19 **Injections**

A patient is given flucloxacillin 800 mg, IV. The drug is available in vials containing 1 g in 5 mL. How much of the drug will be discarded?

20 **Injections**

A patient has been prescribed 4 mg morphine IM. The drug is available in a 10 mL pre-filled syringe containing 1 mg morphine/mL. How many millilitres of morphine should be discarded?

21 **Intravenous infusions**

A patient is to receive 0.9% saline by IV infusion. The flow rate is set to deliver 90 mL/h. How much fluid will the patient receive over 3 h?

22 **Intravenous infusions**

A patient is given an IV infusion of penicillin. The flow rate is set at 120 mL/h. After 6 h, how much has the patient received?

23 **Intravenous infusions**

Hartmann's solution is administered to a patient IV at a rate of 125 mL/h. How much will the patient receive over 20 h?

24 **Intravenous infusions**

A patient is to receive 100 mL of normal saline, IV. If the pump is set at 150 mL/h, how long will the infusion take?

25 **Intravenous infusions**

How long will a 750 mL infusion, given at a flow rate of 250 mL/h, take to deliver?

26 **Intravenous infusions**

How long will a 1 L infusion take if the infusion pump is set to deliver 200 mL/h?

27 **Intravenous infusions**

What is the required flow rate if a patient is to be given a 150 mL infusion of normal saline over 3 h?

28 **Intravenous infusions**

Over a period of 10 h, a patient is to receive 1 L of chemotherapy. What should the flow rate of the infusion pump be set at?

29 **Intravenous infusions**

A patient is to be given an IV infusion of normal saline over 2 h. The infusion begins at 14.15 hours. What time should the infusion stop?

30 **Intravenous infusions**

An older patient suffering from dehydration is put on an IV infusion over 6 h. The infusion begins at 09.10 hours. What time does the infusion stop?

31 **Parenteral feeding**

A patient is to be given a 720 mL infusion of parenteral feed supplement over 24 h. Calculate the flow rate.

32 | Parenteral feeding

A patient with severe burns trauma has been prescribed 0.8 L supplemental parenteral nutrition by intravenous infusion. The flow rate is set at 40 mL/h. How long should the infusion run?

33 | Parenteral feeding

A patient is to receive a 1200 mL PEG feed over 8 h. What is the required flow rate?

34 | Parenteral feeding

Feeding over 6 h via PEG tubing has been prescribed for a patient with oesophageal problems. If the feed is commenced at 16.30 hours, with a 1 h break at 19.00 hours, at what time will the feed be complete?

35 | Parenteral feeding

An undernourished patient is to be administered total intravenous nutrition prior to undergoing radiation therapy. The 1 L infusion volume is to be administered at a rate of 125 mL/h. If the infusion starts at 08.30 hours, what time will it finish?

36 | Paediatric drugs

A child weighing 16 kg is prescribed erythromycin in 4 divided doses. The recommended maximum dose is 40 mg/kg/day. How much erythromycin is given in a single dose?

37 | Paediatric drugs

Benzylpenicillin sodium is to be administered to a child. The prescribed dose is 100 mg/kg/day in 4 divided doses. If the child weighs 12 kg, calculate the size of a single dose.

38 | Paediatric drugs

A child is to be given cefalexin at a dose of 30 mg/kg/day in 3 divided doses. How much drug should be administered in a single dose, given that the child weighs 9 kg?

39 **Paediatric drugs**

Amoxicillin is prescribed for a child weighing 20 kg at a dose of 45 mg/kg/day, to be taken in 4 divided doses. What is the size of a single dose?

40 **Paediatric drugs**

Chloramphenicol is to be administered at the recommended dose of 40 mg/kg/day in 4 divided doses to a child weighing 25 kg. Calculate the size of a single dose.

1 **Oral medication**
2 tablets

2 **Oral medication**
$\frac{1}{2}$ tablet

3 **Oral medication**
$\frac{1}{2}$ tablet

4 **Oral medication**
3 tablets

5 **Oral medication**
2 tablets

6 **Oral medication**
5 tablets

7 **Oral medication**
a. 250 mg   b. 375 mg   c. 500 mg

8 **Oral medication**
a. 400 mg   b. 600 mg   c. 1000 mg

9 **Oral medication**
a. 375 mg   b. 500 mg   c. 750 mg

10 **Oral medication**
  a. 62.5 mg   b. 312.5 mg   c. 625 mg

11 **Oral medication**
  5 mL

12 **Oral medication**
  15 mL

13 **Oral medication**
  10 mL

14 **Oral medication**
  16 mL

15 **Oral medication**
  5 mL

16 **Injections**
  2.5 mL

17 **Injections**
  0.5 mL

18 **Injections**
  2.4 mL

19 **Injections**
  1 mL

20 **Injections**
  6 mL

21 **Intravenous infusions**
  270 mL

22 **Intravenous infusions**
  720 mL

23 **Intravenous infusions**
  2.5 L

24 **Intravenous infusions**
  40 minutes

25 **Intravenous infusions**
  3 h

26 **Intravenous infusions**
  5 h

27 **Intravenous infusions**
  50 mL/h

28 **Intravenous infusions**
  100 mL/h

29 **Intravenous infusions**
  16.15 hours

30 **Intravenous infusion**
  15.10 hours

31 **Parenteral feeding**
  30 mL/h

32 **Parenteral feeding**
  20 h

33 **Parenteral feeding**
  150 mL/h

34   **Parenteral feeding**
      23.30 hours

35   **Parenteral feeding**
      16.30 hours

36   **Paediatric drugs**
      160 mg

37   **Paediatric drugs**
      300 mg

38   **Paediatric drugs**
      90 mg

39   **Paediatric drugs**
      225 mg

40   **Paediatric drugs**
      250 mg

12 Oral medication

The most common way of administering medication is to give it by mouth (orally). This route offers several benefits to the patient: it is usually easy to administer, it is not invasive, and it normally does not cause pain.

Furthermore, specialized equipment is not usually needed and most patients can readily self-administer.

For administering tablets and capsules, the most useful equation is:

$$\text{Number required} = \frac{\text{Amount prescribed}}{\text{Amount in each tablet or capsule}}$$

WORKED EXAMPLE: TABLETS

Calculate the following:

A patient is prescribed 1 g paracetamol orally. The medication is available in 500 mg tablets. How many tablets should be administered?

STEP 1

Identify the equation that you need.

$$\text{Number required} = \frac{\text{Amount prescribed}}{\text{Amount in each tablet or capsule}}$$

STEP 2

Check the units of weight, and convert as necessary so that the amount prescribed and the amount in each tablet are expressed in the same units. Substitute the appropriate terms in the equation with the relevant values. In this case the amount prescribed is 1 g, which is 1000 mg, and the stock amount available is 500 mg.

$$\text{Number required} = \frac{1000 \text{ mg}}{500 \text{ mg}}$$

STEP 3

To simplify the equation, divide the numerator (the top line) by the denominator (the bottom line).

$$\text{Number required} = \frac{\cancel{1000}^{2} \text{ mg}}{\cancel{500}_{1} \text{ mg}}$$

$$= \frac{2}{1}$$

$$= 2 \text{ tablets}$$

The answer is   **2 tablets**

For liquid medications and suspensions, a variation of the same equation is used.

$$\text{Volume required} = \frac{\text{Strength prescribed}}{\text{Strength available}} \times \text{Volume of stock}$$

WORKED EXAMPLE: LIQUIDS AND SUSPENSIONS

Calculate the following:

A patient is prescribed 250 mg penicillin orally. The medication is available as a syrup, 500 mg in 5 mL. What volume of suspension should the patient be given?

STEP 1

Identify the equation you need.

$$\text{Volume required} = \frac{\text{Strength prescribed}}{\text{Strength available}} \times \text{Volume of stock}$$

STEP 2

Check the units of weight and convert as necessary. Substitute the appropriate terms with the relevant values. In this case the strength prescribed is 250 mg, and the strength available is 500 mg. (These are both expressed in milligrams, so no conversion is necessary.) The stock volume is 5 mL.

$$\text{Volume required} = \frac{250 \text{ mg}}{500 \text{ mg}} \times 5 \text{ mL}$$

STEP 3

To simplify the equation, divide the numerator (the top line) by the denominator (the bottom line). In this case, the denominator is larger than the numerator: dividing 250 by 500 gives ½. Alternatively, we could consider this as dividing the denominator by the numerator. (What we are actually doing is dividing both the numerator and the denominator by their highest common factor, which in this case is 250.)

$$\text{Volume required} = \frac{\overset{1}{\cancel{250}} \text{ mg}}{\underset{2}{\cancel{500}} \text{ mg}} \times 5 \text{ mL}$$

$$= \frac{1}{2} \times 5 \text{ mL}$$

$$= 2.5 \text{ mL}$$

The answer is **2.5 mL**

CHECK-UP TEST: ORAL MEDICATION

Calculate the following:

a. A patient is prescribed 2 g flucloxacillin to be taken orally. The drug is available in 500 mg capsules. How many should be given?

b. Chlorambucil is prescribed for a patient at a dose of 8 mg a day. The tablets are available in 2 mg doses. How many tablets should the patient receive over 24 h?

c. A patient is prescribed paroxetine 40 mg daily in two divided doses. The tablets are available in 20 mg tablets. How many should the patient be given per dose?

d. An older patient is to be given 500 mg paracetamol, which is available from stock as a 250 mg/5 mL suspension. What volume should the patient be given?

e. Pethidine 25 mg has been prescribed for a patient. The pharmacy stocks a multidose vial containing 50 mg/mL. How many millilitres should you administer?

f. A patient requires 20 mmol of potassium chloride oral solution. The solution contains 80 mmol in every 20 mL. What volume should you give the patient?

ANSWERS

a. 4 capsules   b. 4 tablets   c. 1 tablet

d. 10 mL   e. 0.5 mL   f. 5 mL

13 Injections

There are many reasons for giving medications by injection. Some are given subcutaneously (under the skin) because they cannot be absorbed readily from the stomach or intestinal mucosa. Others may be labile (unstable), or easily broken down by digestive enzymes. Intramuscular injections may be given for patients who require inoculations, post-operative analgesics or anti-emetics, and medications for patients who may not tolerate IV infusions.

The administration of medication by injection has become less common in recent times. Subcutaneous and intramuscular injections are both painful, and some medications may be traumatic to tissue. Many drugs that were previously given by injection are now given by IV infusion.

The equation that is of most use for calculating injection volumes is similar to that used in Chapter 12 for oral suspensions and liquids.

$$\text{Volume required} = \frac{\text{Strength prescribed}}{\text{Strength available}} \times \text{Volume of stock}$$

WORKED EXAMPLE: INJECTIONS

Calculate the following:

A patient has been prescribed 6000 units of dalteparin sodium to be given subcutaneously. The available drug comes in a vial containing 10000 units/mL. What volume should be given?

STEP 1

Identify the equation that you need.

$$\text{Volume required} = \frac{\text{Strength prescribed}}{\text{Strength available}} \times \text{Volume of stock}$$

STEP 2

Check the units. Substitute the appropriate terms with the relevant values. In this case the strength prescribed is 6000 units, and the strength available is 10000 units per millilitre. The stock volume is 1 mL.

$$\text{Volume required} = \frac{6000 \text{ mg}}{10000 \text{ mg}} \times 1 \text{ mL}$$

STEP 3

Simplify the equation as shown below.

$$\text{Volume required} = \frac{\cancel{6000}^{\,3} \text{ mg}}{\cancel{10000}_{5} \text{ mg}} \times 1 \text{ mL}$$

$$= \frac{3}{5} \times 1 \text{ mL}$$

$$= 0.6 \text{ mL}$$

The answer is **0.6 mL**

CHECK-UP TEST: INJECTIONS

Calculate the following:

a. A patient has been prescribed 10 units of regular insulin. The ampoule is labelled 100 units/mL. What injection volume should the patient receive?

b. Morphine sulphate 10 mg has been prescribed for your patient, and is available in a vial containing 20 mg/mL. How many millilitres of the drug should be administered?

c. A diabetic patient is prescribed 45 units of insulin daily. The insulin is available as 100 units/mL. How much should be injected?

d. A patient is prescribed benzylpenicillin sodium 800 mg. The available concentration is 1.2 g in 6 mL. How much should be drawn up for injection?

e. Tramadol hydrochloride 80 mg is required. Available is 100 mg in 2 mL. How much needs to be drawn up from the vial?

f. Erythromycin 250 mg is prescribed. Available from stock is a concentration of 1 g in 10 mL. How much is required to be drawn up?

ANSWERS

d. 4 mL	e. 1.6 mL	f. 2.5 mL
a. 0.1 mL	b. 0.5 mL	c. 0.45 mL

14 Intravenous infusions

The careful administration of IV fluids is critical when dealing with patients who are susceptible to fluid volume changes. Rapid infusion of IV fluids or blood product may threaten the patient's well-being, and therefore the flow rate should be closely monitored.

The flow rate is generally defined as the '*number of millilitres of fluid to be administered over 1 hour*' (although it can also refer to the number of millilitres to be delivered over a minute).

Normally the flow of an infusion is regulated by means of an electronic infusion device. These automatic devices generally require programming, and should be checked using the formula below.

$$\text{Flow rate (mL/h)} = \frac{\text{Volume of infusion}}{\text{Number of hours to run}}$$

WORKED EXAMPLE: AUTOMATIC INFUSIONS

Calculate the following:

A patient has been prescribed 2000 mL of fluid over 24 hours. What is the flow rate?

STEP 1

Identify the equation you need.

$$\text{Flow rate (mL/h)} = \frac{\text{Volume of infusion}}{\text{Number of hours to run}}$$

STEP 2

Check the units. Substitute the appropriate terms with the relevant values. In this case the volume prescribed is 2000 mL, and the time to run is 24 h.

$$\text{Flow rate (mL/h)} = \frac{2000 \text{ mL}}{24 \text{ h}}$$

STEP 3

Simplify the equation by dividing the numerator (the top line) by the denominator (the bottom line).

$$\text{Flow rate (mL/h)} = \frac{\cancel{2000}^{83.3} \text{ mL}}{\cancel{24}_{1} \text{ h}}$$

$$= \frac{83.3}{1}$$

$$= 83.3 \text{ mL}$$

Usually this would be rounded down to 83 mL.

The answer is **83 mL**

In certain situations automatic pumps may not be available, and infusions or fluid replacement therapy must be administered by a manual infusion under the influence of gravity. To set up a manual infusion accurately, the number of drops per minute must be calculated. This depends on the volume to be infused in terms of drops, which in turn is related to the characteristics of the giving set used in the infusion.

Standard giving sets are either *macro-drip sets*, with a drip factor of 20 drops/mL (or 15 drops/mL for blood), or *micro-drip sets*, with a drip factor of 60 drops/mL. Macro-drip sets are used in situations that require infusions of large volumes. Micro-drip sets are used to administer smaller volumes, and in situations where greater accuracy may be required.

The standard formula for checking manual infusions is given below.

$$\text{Drip rate (drops/min)} = \frac{\text{Drops/mL of the giving set} \times \text{Volume}}{\text{Number of hours to run} \times 60}$$

WORKED EXAMPLE: MANUAL INFUSIONS

Calculate the drip rate required to administer an infusion of 750 mL of 0.9% sodium chloride over 6 hours using a macro-drip giving set (20 drops/min).

STEP 1

Identify the equation you need.

$$\text{Drip rate (drops/min)} = \frac{\text{Drops/mL of the giving set} \times \text{Volume}}{\text{Number of hours to run} \times 60}$$

STEP 2

Check the units, and the drip factor of the giving set. Convert the required volume to the equivalent number of drops by multiplying the volume of infusion by the drip factor. In this case the volume prescribed is 750 mL, and the drip factor of the giving set is 20 drops/mL. Substitute these values into the top line of the fraction (the numerator).

$$\text{Drip rate (drops/min)} = \frac{20 \text{ drops/mL} \times 750 \text{ mL}}{\text{Number of hours to run} \times 60}$$

STEP 3

In the bottom line of the fraction (the denominator), convert the time the infusion has to run (the number of hours) to minutes by multiplying by 60. For part hours remember to add on the relevant number of minutes.

$$\text{Drip rate (drops/min)} = \frac{20 \text{ drops/mL} \times 750 \text{ mL}}{6 \times 60}$$

STEP 4

Multiply out the numerator (notice how the mL units cancel out) and the denominator, and then simplify the equation by dividing the numerator (the top number) by the denominator (the bottom number).

$$\text{Drip rate (drops/min)} = \frac{20 \times 750}{6 \times 60}$$

$$= \frac{15000}{360}$$

$$= \frac{\cancel{15000}^{41.7}}{\cancel{360}_{1}}$$

$$= \frac{41.7}{1}$$

$$= 41.7 \text{ drops/min}$$

As you cannot give a fraction of a drop, this would normally be rounded up to 42 drops/min.

The answer is **42 drops/min**

 CHECK-UP TEST: INTRAVENOUS INFUSIONS

Calculate the following:

a. A 1000 mL infusion of glucose 5% in water is given over 5 hours. What is the hourly flow rate?

b. A patient is to receive 1 g vancomycin in 200 mL over 4 hours. Calculate the flow hourly flow rate.

c. Ceftriaxone, 2 g in 500 mL water over 10 hours, is prescribed. What is the hourly flow rate?

d. Ifosfamide, 2 g in 0.9% sodium chloride is given over 24 hours. The total volume of infusion is 3 L. What is the hourly flow rate?

e. A patient requires a continuous infusion of 25000 units of heparin in 500 mL in normal saline. If the patient receives 750 units/hour, what is the flow rate?

f. Lidocaine, 1 g in 250 mL of fluid, is prescribed, and is to infuse at a rate of 3 mg/min. What is the flow rate?

g. Calculate the drip rate for a 1250 mL infusion of 5% glucose in water over 12 hours using a macro-drip set (20 drops/mL).

h. A patient is to receive 1.5 L of fluid over 13 hours using a macro-drip set (20 drops/mL). Calculate the drip rate.

i. A 400 mL infusion of flucloxacillin is to be administered over 6 hours using a macro-drip set (20 drops/mL). What should the drip rate be set at?

j. A transfusion of packed cells is requested for an anaemic patient over 3 hours. The volume of packed cells is 250 mL. The giving set delivers 15 drops/mL. Calculate the drip rate.

k. A child is prescribed 60 mL infusion over 2 hours. The micro-drip set delivers 60 drops/mL. What is the correct drip rate for this patient?

l. An infant is prescribed a 180 mL infusion of flucytosine over 5 hours using a micro-drip set (60 drops/mL). Determine the correct drip rate.

ANSWERS

j. 21 drops/min

k. 30 drops/min

l. 36 drops/min

g. 35 drops/min

h. 38 drops/min

i. 22 drops/min

d. 125 mL/h

e. 15 mL/h

f. 45 mL/h

a. 200 mL/h

b. 50 mL/h

c. 50 mL/h

15 Parenteral nutrition

Parenteral nutrition is administered to a patient when their nutritional requirements cannot be met because of increased metabolic demand, or because of impaired digestion or absorption processes.

The procedure involves administering commercially available products or specially formulated pharmacy preparations. This might be via a central or peripheral vein, but in most cases nutrients are delivered directly to the gastrointestinal tract by means of a percutaneous endoscopic gastrostomy (PEG) tube.

The flow of PEG feeding is normally controlled by an automated infusion pump. These automatic devices are similar to those used for drug infusions, whereby a pre-determined flow rate can be set.

To check that the infusion is not or has not been administered at too fast a rate, it is important to be able to determine the finish time, given the start time and the flow rate.

The basic formula is given below.

$$\text{Protocol time (hours)} = \frac{\text{Volume of infusion}}{\text{Flow rate}}$$

If the infusion has to run for a significant number of hours, a break may be incorporated into the protocol. The length of this break must be added to the above formula to give the actual finish time.

$$\text{Protocol time (hours)} = \frac{\text{Volume of infusion}}{\text{Flow rate}} + \text{Break time}$$

WORKED EXAMPLE: PARENTERAL NUTRITION

Calculate the following:

A patient has been prescribed 900 mL parenteral nutrition to be administered by PEG tube at a flow rate of 150 mL/h. The infusion is scheduled to start at 07.30 hours with a 2 h break mid-infusion. What time will the feed be completed?

STEP 1

Identify the equation you need.

$$\text{Protocol time (hours)} = \frac{\text{Volume of infusion}}{\text{Flow rate}} + \text{Break time}$$

STEP 2

Substitute the volume of infusion (900 mL), flow rate (150 mL/h) and break time (2 h) into the equation and then simplify.

$$\text{Protocol time} = \frac{900 \text{ mL}}{150 \text{ mL/h}} + 2 \text{ hours}$$

$$= \frac{900^6}{150_1} + 2 \text{ hours}$$

$$= 6 + 2 \text{ hours}$$

$$= 8 \text{ hours}$$

STEP 3

To determine the time at which the infusion should be terminated, add the protocol time to the start time.

$$\text{Finish time} = \text{Start time} + \text{Protocol time}$$

In this case the protocol time is 8 hours and the start time is 07.30 hours.

$$\text{Finish time} = 07.30 \text{ hours} + 8 \text{ hours}$$

$$= 15.30 \text{ hours}$$

The answer is **15.30 hours**

 # CHECK-UP TEST: PARENTERAL NUTRITION

Calculate the following:

a. Parenteral nutrition (450 mL) is to be given to a patient over 3 hours. What is the correct flow rate?

b. A patient has been prescribed a 1200 mL PEG feed at a flow rate of 120 mL/h. The infusion is scheduled to start at 09.30 hours with a 1 hour break during the infusion. What time will the feed be completed?

c. A PEG feed is to be administered at a flow rate of 50 mL/h. The volume to be given is 600 mL. A 2 h break from the infusion has been indicated. The protocol is scheduled to commence at 08.00 hours. At what time will the feed be complete?

d. A parenteral infusion supplement (500 mL) is prescribed for an older patient over a 4 h period. The protocol initially requires a flow rate of 50 mL/h for 90 min. What should the flow rate be increased to if the protocol is to finish on schedule?

e. A flow rate of 125 mL/h is used to administer a 1.5 L PEG feed to a patient awaiting chemotherapy. The protocol starts at 09.30 hours. A break is scheduled from 13.00 to 14.30 hours. What time will the infusion be complete?

f. A patient is prescribed a 1.2 L PEG feed. The protocol is scheduled to commence at 10.30 hours at a flow rate of 125 mL/h. After 4 hours the procedure is stopped for a 2 hour break and then recommenced at a flow rate of 200 mL/h. What time will the protocol finish?

ANSWERS

a. 150 mL/h

b. 20.30 hours

c. 22.00 hours

d. 170 mL/h

e. 23.00 hours

f. 20.00 hours

16 Paediatric drugs

The administration of drugs to paediatric patients is a complex and specialist area. It is based primarily on body weight, although certain drugs may be administered on the basis of body surface area. This chapter focuses on medications administered on the basis of body weight.

The basic calculation depends on an accurate determination of the child's weight, but remember that before a dose is prescribed for an infant or child, the appropriateness of their weight for their age and height need to be assessed. This is especially pertinent given the increasing incidence of obesity in infants and young children.

Marked differences in the distribution, metabolism and therapeutic index (TI) of drugs in adults and children mean that extreme caution should be taken when prescribing or administering drugs to children, as even the most insignificant of errors can be potentially life-threatening.

Many pharmaceutical companies provide clinical trials data relating to safe drug dosages for paediatric patients in milligrams per kilogram (mg/kg) of body weight. Based on this information, the paediatric dose can be determined by multiplying the weight of the patient (in kilograms) by the prescribed number of milligrams of drug per kilogram (which may be reported per dose or per day).

Dose required = Body weight (kg) × Recommended dose (mg/kg/day)

WORKED EXAMPLE: PAEDIATRIC DRUGS

Calculate the following:

A 6-year-old patient has been prescribed erythromycin by continuous infusion at a dose of 50 mg/kg/day. The child weighs 24 kg. What dose should be administered?

STEP 1

Identify the equation you need.

Dose required = Body weight (kg) × Recommended dose (mg/kg/day)

STEP 2

Substitute the patient's body weight (24 kg) and the recommended dose (50 mg/kg/day) into the equation.

$$\text{Dose required} = 24 \text{ kg} \times 50 \text{ mg/kg/day}$$

$$= 1200 \text{ mg}$$

The answer is **1200 mg**

 CHECK-UP TEST: PAEDIATRIC DRUGS

Calculate the following:

a. The suggested paediatric dose for a drug is 75 mg/kg/day. How much should a child weighing 30 kg be prescribed?

b. An infant weighing 16 kg has been prescribed 150 mg/kg/day of an antibiotic to be administered by IV injection, in 4 divided doses. What dose should be administered in each injection?

c. Calculate the size of a single dose for an 18 kg child prescribed chloramphenicol 40 mg/kg/day in 3 divided doses.

d. A 13 kg child is prescribed 80 mg/kg/day ampicillin in 4 divided doses. Calculate the size of a single dose.

e. A 7-year-old child weighing 24 kg is prescribed a potent antibiotic for a severe infection. The drug is to be administered at a dose of 75 mg/kg every 8 hours. What is the total daily dose?

f. A 9 kg child has been prescribed amoxicillin (25 mg/kg/day) to be given in equally divided doses every 8 hours. How much antibiotic should be administered in each dose?

ANSWERS

<table>
<tr><td>d. 260 mg</td><td>e. 5400 mg</td><td>f. 75 mg</td></tr>
<tr><td>a. 2250 mg</td><td>b. 600 mg</td><td>c. 240 mg</td></tr>
</table>

QUESTIONS

FOR EACH OF THE FOLLOWING CALCULATE THE CORRECT ANSWER

1 | **Oral medication**

A patient is prescribed 1.5 g paracetamol by mouth. Stock is available in 500 mg tablets. How many tablets should be given?

2 | **Oral medication**

A patient is prescribed 20 mg temazepam. Stock available from the pharmacy comes in 10 mg tablets. How many tablets should be administered?

3 | **Oral medication**

Sodium valproate is prescribed for a patient at a dose of 100 micrograms. The medication is available as 0.2 mg tablets. How many should be given?

4 | **Oral medication**

1 g of ampicillin is prescribed. The stock available comes in 250 mg capsules. How many should be given?

5 | **Oral medication**

A patient is to receive 8 mg of fesoterodine. 4 mg tablets are available. How many should the patient be given?

6 | **Oral medication**

A patient requires 12 mg tizanidine. Tablets are available in 4 mg doses. How many should the patient be given?

7 | **Oral medication**

A suspension contains cefadroxil 250 mg/5 mL. How many milligrams of the drug are contained in each of the following volumes?

    a.   10 mL   b.   15 mL   c. 20 mL

8 | **Oral medication**

Methadone hydrochloride is available as a solution containing 5 mg/mL. How many milligrams of medication are contained in the following volumes?

    a.   2.5 mL   b.   5 mL   c. 10 mL

9 | **Oral medication**

Amitriptyline hydrochloride is available as a solution containing 25 mg/5 mL. How much of the drug is contained in the following volumes?

    a.   7.5 mL   b.   10 mL   c. 15 mL

10 | **Oral medication**

A syrup contains 15 mg/mL of lacosamide. How much of the drug is contained in each of the following volumes?

    a.   2.5 mL   b.   5 mL   c. 7.5 mL

11 | **Oral medication**

A patient is prescribed flucloxacillin, 400 mg to be given orally. The suspension contains 250 mg/5 mL. How much should be given?

12 | **Oral medication**

A patient is prescribed 500000 units of nystatin by mouth. A stock suspension is available as 100000 units/mL. How much should be given?

13 **Oral medication**

Phenoxymethylpenicillin suspension 750 mg is to be given to a patient. The stock contains 250 mg in 5 mL. What volume should be given?

14 **Oral medication**

Abacavir 150 mg is prescribed. A solution containing 20 mg/mL is available. What volume should be dispensed?

15 **Oral medication**

Oseltamivir is to be given at a dose of 75 mg daily. Available stock is 60 mg/mL. What volume should be given?

16 **Injections**

Sodium valproate 400 mg is to be administered by slow injection. The medication is available in vials containing 100 mg/mL. How much should be drawn up for injection?

17 **Injections**

Bemiparin sodium, a low molecular weight heparin, is available at a strength of 12500 units/mL. A patient is prescribed 2500 units. How much should be drawn up for injection?

18 **Injections**

A patient is to receive an injection of 750 mg ampicillin. The drug is available in ampoules containing 500 mg/mL. How much is required for injection?

19 **Injections**

A patient is given ceftriaxone 250 mg, IV. The drug is available in vials containing 1 g in 4 mL. How much of the drug will be discarded?

20 **Injections**

A patient has been prescribed 450 units of follitropin alpha. The drug is available in a pre-filled syringe containing 600 units/mL. How much of the preparation should be discarded?

21 Intravenous infusions

A patient is to receive 0.9% saline by IV infusion. The flow rate is set to deliver 75 mL/h. How much fluid will the patient receive over 5 h?

22 Intravenous infusions

A patient is given an IV infusion of penicillin. The flow rate is set at 125 mL/h. After 6 h, what volume has the patient received?

23 Intravenous infusions

Hartmann's solution is administered to a patient IV at a rate of 150 mL/h. How much will the patient receive over 20 h?

24 Intravenous infusions

A patient is to receive 200 mL of normal saline, IV. If the pump is set at 150 mL/h, how long will the infusion take?

25 Intravenous infusions

How long will a 1500 mL infusion, given at a flow rate of 250 mL/h, take to deliver?

26 Intravenous infusions

How long will a 1 L infusion take if the infusion pump is set to deliver 150 mL/h?

27 Intravenous infusions

What is the required flow rate if a patient is to be given a 240 mL infusion of normal saline over 3 h?

28 Intravenous infusions

Over a period of 5 hours, a patient is to receive 1 L of chemotherapy. What should the flow rate of the infusion pump be set at?

29 Intravenous infusions

A patient is to be given an IV infusion of 600 mL normal saline over 3 h. The infusion begins at 14.15 hours. What time should the infusion stop?

30 **Intravenous infusions**

An older patient suffering from dehydration is put on an IV infusion over 4 hours. The infusion begins at 09.10 hours. What time does the infusion stop?

31 **Parenteral nutrition**

Determine the time taken for delivery of a parenteral feed supplement (450 mL) given at a flow rate of 150 mL/h.

32 **Parenteral nutrition**

A patient awaiting chemotherapy has been prescribed 1 L of parenteral nutrition by PEG tubing. The flow rate is set at 100 mL/h. How long should the infusion run?

33 **Parenteral nutrition**

A 900 mL PEG feed is prescribed for a patient, and is to be administered over 6 hours. What is the required flow rate?

34 **Parenteral nutrition**

A malnourished patient with oesophageal varices has been prescribed a nutritional supplement by parenteral infusion. If the protocol is commenced at 13.00 hours and lasts for 300 minutes, at what time will the protocol finish?

35 **Parenteral nutrition**

A patient is prescribed a 1 L PEG feed to be administered at a flow rate of 100 mL/h. If the protocol begins at 07.00 hours and a break of 30 minutes is incorporated into the procedure, what time will the protocol finish?

36 **Paediatric drugs**

A child weighing 18 kg is prescribed erythromycin in 3 divided doses. The recommended maximum dose is 40 mg/kg/day. How much erythromycin is given in a single dose?

37 **Paediatric drugs**

Ibuprofen is to be administered to a child. The recommended dose is 30 mg/kg/day in 3 divided doses. If the child weighs 10 kg, calculate the size of a single dose.

38 Paediatric drugs

A child is to be given cefalexin at a dose of 75 mg/kg/day in 3 divided doses. How much drug should be administered in a single dose, given that the child weighs 15 kg?

39 Paediatric drugs

Amoxicillin is prescribed for a child weighing 20 kg at a dose of 50 mg/kg/day to be taken in 4 divided doses. What is the size of a single dose?

40 Paediatric drugs

Chlorpromazine hydrochloride is to be administered to a child weighing 20 kg. The recommended dose is 1.5 mg/kg/day in 3 divided doses. Calculate the size of a single dose.

ANSWERS

1 **Oral medication**
3 tablets

2 **Oral medication**
2 tablets

3 **Oral medication**

$\frac{1}{2}$ tablet

4 **Oral medication**
4 tablets

5 **Oral medication**
2 tablets

6 **Oral medication**
3 tablets

7 **Oral medication**
a. 500 mg b. 750 mg c. 1000 mg

8 **Oral medication**
a. 12.5 mg b. 25 mg c. 50 mg

9 **Oral medication**
a. 37.5 mg b. 50 mg c. 75 mg

10 **Oral medication**
    a.   37.5 mg   b.   75 mg   c. 112.5 mg

11 **Oral medication**
    8 mL

12 **Oral medication**
    5 mL

13 **Oral medication**
    15 mL

14 **Oral medication**
    7.5 mL

15 **Oral medication**
    1.25 mL

16 **Injections**
    4 mL

17 **Injections**
    0.2 mL

18 **Injections**
    1.5 mL

19 **Injections**
    3 mL

20 **Injections**
    0.25 mL

21 **Intravenous infusions**
375 mL

22 **Intravenous infusions**
750 mL

23 **Intravenous infusions**
3000 mL

24 **Intravenous infusions**
1 h 20 min

25 **Intravenous infusions**
6 h

26 **Intravenous infusions**
6 h 40 min

27 **Intravenous infusions**
80 mL/h

28 **Intravenous infusions**
200 mL/h

29 **Intravenous infusions**
17.15 hours

30 **Intravenous infusion**
13.10 hours

31 **Parenteral nutrition**
3 hours

32   **Parenteral nutrition**
10 hours

33   **Parenteral nutrition**
150 mL/h

34   **Parenteral nutrition**
18.00 hours

35   **Parenteral nutrition**
17.30 hours

36   **Paediatric drugs**
240 mg

37   **Paediatric drugs**
100 mg

38   **Paediatric drugs**
375 mg

39   **Paediatric drugs**
250 mg

40   **Paediatric drugs**
10 mg

SECTION C
Appendices

1 Useful mathematical terms

Decimal fraction: Fraction in which the denominator is a multiple of 10.

Denominator: The bottom number in a fraction, which represents the total number of equal parts of a whole number.

Dividend: In division, the number to be divided.

Divisor: In division, the number by which the dividend is divided.

Factor: A number that will divide into another number exactly. For example, the factors of 10 are 1, 2 and 5.

Fraction: A number that represents a part of a whole number.

Improper fraction: Fraction in which the numerator is greater than the denominator.

Lowest common denominator: Smallest number that is a multiple of all denominators in a series of fractions.

Mixed number: Number that consists of a whole number and a fraction.

Numerator: The top number in a fraction, which represents the number of equal parts represented by the fraction.

Percentage: Number of parts of a quantity per hundred.

Product: The answer of a multiplication problem.

Proper fraction: Fraction in which the numerator is less than the denominator.

Quotient: The answer of a division problem.

Rounding: Reducing the number of decimal places used to express a number.

Common units of measurement

Metric weight

1 kilogram (kg)	= 1000 grams (g)
1 g	= 1000 milligrams (mg)
1 mg	= 1000 micrograms (mcg)

0.1 g	= 100 mg
0.01 g	= 10 mg
0.001 g	= 1 mg

Metric volume

1 litre (L)	= 1000 millilitres (mL)
1 mL	= 1000 microlitres

0.1 L	= 100 mL
0.01 L	= 10 mL
0.001 L	= 1 mL

3 Formulae used in this book

Oral Medications

Tablets and capsules

$$\text{Number required} = \frac{\text{Amount prescribed}}{\text{Amount in each tablet or capsule}}$$

Liquids and suspensions

$$\text{Volume required} = \frac{\text{Strength prescribed}}{\text{Strength available}} \times \text{Volume of stock}$$

Injections

$$\text{Volume required} = \frac{\text{Strength prescribed}}{\text{Strength available}} \times \text{Volume of stock}$$

Infusions

Automatic

$$\text{Flow rate (mL/h)} = \frac{\text{Volume of infusion}}{\text{Number of hours to run}}$$

Manual

$$\text{Drip rate (drops/min)} = \frac{\text{Drops/mL of the giving set} \times \text{Volume}}{\text{Number of hours to run} \times 60}$$

Parenteral Infusions

$$\text{Protocol time (hours)} = \frac{\text{Volume of infusion}}{\text{Flow rate}} + \text{Break time}$$

Paediatric Drugs

$$\text{Dose required} = \text{Body weight (kg)} \times \text{Recommended dose (mg/kg/day)}$$

4 Multiplication chart

	1	2	3	4	5	6	7	8	9	10	11	12
1	1	2	3	4	5	6	7	8	9	10	11	12
2	2	4	6	8	10	12	14	16	18	20	22	24
3	3	6	9	12	15	18	21	24	27	30	33	36
4	4	8	12	16	20	24	28	32	36	40	44	48
5	5	10	15	20	25	30	35	40	45	50	55	60
6	6	12	18	24	30	36	42	48	54	60	66	72
7	7	14	21	28	35	42	49	56	63	70	77	84
8	8	16	24	32	40	48	56	64	72	80	88	96
9	9	18	27	36	45	54	63	72	81	90	99	108
10	10	20	30	40	50	60	70	80	90	100	110	120
11	11	22	33	44	55	66	77	88	99	110	121	132
12	12	24	36	48	60	72	84	96	108	120	132	144

5 Selected references

Brown, M., and Mulholland, J.L. *Drug Calculations: Process and Problems for Clinical Practice*, 8th ed. St Louis: Mosby/Elsevier, 2008.

Downie, G., Mackenzie, J., and Williams A. *Pharmacology and Medicines Management for Nurses*, 4th ed. Edinburgh: Churchill Livingstone, 2008.

Gould, D., and Greenstein, B. *Trounce's Clinical Pharmacology for Nurses*, 18th ed. Edinburgh: Churchill Livingstone, 2009.

Gray Morris, D.C. *Calculate with Confidence*, 5th ed. St Louis: Mosby/Elsevier, 2010.

Greengold, N.L., et al. 'The impact of dedicated medication nurses on the medication administration error rate: a randomized controlled trial', *Archives of Internal Medicine*, vol. 163, no. 19, October 2003, pp. 2359–2367.

Karch, A.M. *Lippincott's Guide to Preventing Medication Errors*. Philadelphia: Lippincott Williams & Wilkins, 2002.

Kee, J.L., and Marshall, S.M. *Clinical Calculations: With Applications to General and Specialty Areas*, 6th ed. Philadelphia: W.B. Saunders, 2008.

Ogden, S.J. *Calculation of Drug Dosages*, 8th ed. St Louis: Mosby/Elsevier, 2007.

Scott, W.N., and McGrath, D. *Dosage Calculations Made Incredibly Easy*. London: Lippincott Williams & Wilkins, 2009.

6 Additional resources

British National Formulary
www.bnf.org

National Institute for Health and Clinical Excellence
www.nice.org.uk

Nursing and Midwifery Council
www.nmc-uk.org

Paediatric Drug Information Advisory Line
www.dial.org.uk
Tel: 0151 252 5837

National Poisons Information Service
www.npis.org
Tel: 0844 892 0111

NURSES! TEST YOURSELF IN PATHOPHYSIOLOGY

Katherine Rogers and William Scott

9780335242238 (Paperback)
April 2011

eBook also available

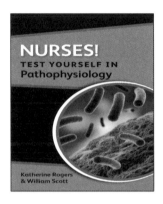

Looking for a quick and effective way to revise and test your knowledge?
This handy book is the essential self-test resource to help nurses revise and prepare for their pathophysiology exams. The book covers a broad range of conditions common to nursing practice including pneumonia, diabetes, asthma, eczema and more. The book includes over 300 questions and 70 glossary terms in total.

Key features:

- Organised into body systems chapters
- Includes a range of question types
- Provides a list of clearly explained answers to questions

www.openup.co.uk

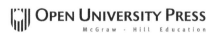

OPEN UNIVERSITY PRESS
McGraw - Hill Education